New Ideas and Techniques in Foot and Ankle Surgery: A Global Perspective

Editors

JOHN G. ANDERSON
DONALD R. BOHAY

FOOT AND ANKLE CLINICS

www.foot.theclinics.com

Consulting Editor
MARK S. MYERSON

June 2016 • Volume 21 • Number 2

ELSEVIER

1600 John F. Kennedy Boulevard • Suite 1800 • Philadelphia, Pennsylvania, 19103-2899

http://www.theclinics.com

FOOT AND ANKLE CLINICS Volume 21, Number 2
June 2016 ISSN 1083-7515, ISBN-13: 978-0-323-41645-0

Editor: Jennifer Flynn-Briggs
Developmental Editor: Meredith Clinton

Foot and Ankle Clinics (ISSN 1083-7515) is published quarterly by Elsevier, Inc., 360 Park Avenue South, New York, NY 10010-1710. Months of issue are March, June, September, and December. Periodicals postage paid at New York, NY, and additional mailing offices. Subscription price per year is $320.00 (US individuals), $466.00 (US institutions), $100.00 (US students), $360.00 (Canadian individuals), $560.00 (Canadian institutions), $215.00 (Canadian students), $460.00 (international individuals), $560.00 (international institutions), and $215.00 (international students). To receive student/resident rate, orders must be accompanied by name of affiliated institution, date of term, and the *signature* of program/residency coordinator on institution letterhead. Orders will be billed at individual rate until proof of status is received. Foreign air speed delivery is included in all *Clinics* subscription prices. All prices are subject to change without notice. **POSTMASTER:** Send address changes to *Foot and Ankle Clinics*, Elsevier Health Sciences Division, Subscription Customer Service, 3251 Riverport Lane, Maryland Heights, MO 63043. **Customer Service: 1-800-654-2452 (US and Canada). From outside of the United States and Canada, call 314-447-8871. Fax: 314-447-8029. E-mail: JournalsCustomerService-usa@ elsevier.com (for print support); JournalsOnlineSupport-usa@elsevier.com (for online support).**

Reprints. For copies of 100 or more, of articles in this publication, please contact the Commercial Reprints Department, Elsevier Inc., 360 Park Avenue South, New York, NY 10010-1710. Tel.: 212-633-3874; Fax: 212-633-3820; E-mail: reprints@elsevier.com.

Contributors

CONSULTING EDITOR

MARK S. MYERSON, MD
Director, Department of Orthopaedic Surgery, The Institute for Foot and Ankle Reconstruction, Mercy Hospital, Mercy Medical Center, Baltimore, Maryland

EDITORS

JOHN G. ANDERSON, MD
Orthopaedic Associates of Michigan; Chairman, Spectrum Health Department of Orthopaedic Surgery; Clinical Professor, Michigan State University College of Human Medicine; Director, GRMEP Orthopaedic Surgery Residency Program; Co-Director, Grand Rapids Orthopaedic Foot and Ankle Fellowship, Grand Rapids, Michigan

DONALD R. BOHAY, MD, FACS
Orthopaedic Associates of Michigan; Clinical Professor, Michigan State University College of Human Medicine; Director, Grand Rapids Orthopaedic Foot and Ankle Fellowship, Grand Rapids, Michigan

AUTHORS

MOSTAFA M. ABOUSAYED, MD
Resident, Department of Orthopedic Surgery, Albany Medical College, Albany, New York; Assistant Lecturer, Department of Orthopedic Surgery, Kasr Al-Ainy Hospital, Cairo University School of Medicine, Cairo, Egypt

DANIEL BAUMFELD, MD
Assistant Professor, Federal University of Minas Gerais, Belo Horizonte, Minas Gerais, Brazil

GREGOR BERRSCHE, MD
ATOS Clinic Heidelberg, Deutsches Gelenkzentrum Heidelberg, Heidelberg, Germany

MICHAEL E. BRAGE, MD
Associate Professor of Orthopaedics, Department of Orthopaedics, University of Washington, Seattle, Washington

MOHAMMED GOMAA, MD
Lecturer, Department of Orthopedic Surgery, Kasr Al-Ainy Hospital, Cairo University School of Medicine, Cairo, Egypt

AMGAD M. HALEEM, MD, PhD
Assistant Professor, Department of Orthopedic Surgery, Oklahoma University College of Medicine Health Sciences Center, Oklahoma City, Oklahoma; Lecturer, Department of Orthopedic Surgery, Kasr Al-Ainy Hospital, Cairo University School of Medicine, Cairo, Egypt

WILLIAM D. HARRISON, MBBS, MRCS, MSc
Foot and Ankle Unit, Royal Liverpool and Broadgreen University Hospitals, Liverpool, United Kingdom

JONAH HEBERT-DAVIES, MD, FRCSC
Associate Professor, Department of Surgery, Université de Montréal, Quebec, Canada; Orthopedic Surgeon, Hôpital du Sacré-Cœur de Montréal, Montréal, Québec, Canada

SEAN WEI LOONG HO, MBBS, MRCS (Edin)
Department of Orthopaedic Surgery, Tan Tock Seng Hospital, Singapore

MICHAEL D. JOHNSON, MD
Assistant Professor of Orthopaedics, Division of Orthopaedics, University of Alabama at Birmingham, Birmingham, Alabama

FABIAN KRAUSE, MD
Department of Orthopaedic Surgery, Inselspital, University of Berne, Berne, Switzerland

WARREN C.W. LATHAM, BScH, MD, FRCSC
Lecturer, University of Toronto; Consultant, University Health Network - Toronto Western Division, Toronto, Ontario, Canada

JOHNNY T.C. LAU, MD, MSc, FRCSC
Orthopaedic Surgeon, Foot and Ankle; Assistant Professor, University of Toronto; Consultant, University Health Network - Toronto Western Division, Toronto, Ontario, Canada

STÉPHANE LEDUC, MD, FRCSC
Associate Professor, Department of Surgery, Université de Montréal, Quebec, Canada; Orthopedic Surgeon, Hôpital du Sacré-Cœur de Montréal, Montréal, Québec, Canada

TRISTAN MEUSNIER, MD
Foot and Ankle Surgery Center, Clinique Saint Charles, Lyon, France

PRIKESHT MUKISH, MD
Foot and Ankle Surgery Center, Clinique Saint Charles, Lyon, France

MARIE-LYNE NAULT, MD, PhD, FRCSC
Associate Professor, Hôpital du Sacré-Coeur de Montréal, Montréal, Québec; Department of Surgery, Université de Montréal, Quebec, Canada; Orthopedic Surgeon, CHU Ste-Justine, Montréal, Québec, Canada

CAIO NERY, MD
Associate Professor, Foot and Ankle Clinic, UNIFESP – Escola Paulista de Medicina, São Paulo, São Paulo, Brazil

CRISTIÁN A. ORTIZ, MD
Foot and Ankle Surgeon, Orthopaedic Department, Clínica Alemana de Santiago, Universidad del Desarrollo, Santiago, Chile

ANNA C. PEAK, FRCS (Orth)
Heatherwood and Wexham Park Hospitals, Ascot, United Kingdom

FERNANDO RADUAN, MD
UNIFESP – Escola Paulista de Medicina, São Paulo, São Paulo, Brazil

DOMINIQUE M. ROULEAU, MD, FRCSC, MSc
Associate Professor, Department of Surgery, Université de Montréal, Quebec, Canada; Orthopedic Surgeon, Hôpital du Sacré-Cœur de Montréal, Montréal, Québec, Canada

TIMO SCHMID, MD
Department of Orthopaedic Surgery, Inselspital, University of Berne, Berne, Switzerland

SEBASTIAN SCHMITT, MD
ATOS Clinic Heidelberg, Deutsches Gelenkzentrum Heidelberg, Heidelberg, Germany

GOWREESON THEVENDRAN, MBChB (Bristol), MFSEM (UK), FRCS Ed (Tr&Orth)
Department of Orthopaedic Surgery, Tan Tock Seng Hospital, Singapore

EMILIO WAGNER, MD
Foot and Ankle Surgeon, Orthopaedic Department, Clínica Alemana de Santiago, Universidad del Desarrollo, Santiago, Chile

PABLO WAGNER, MD
Foot and Ankle Surgeon, Orthopaedic Department, Clínica Alemana de Santiago, Universidad del Desarrollo, Santiago, Chile

CHRISTOPHER R. WALKER, MCh(Orth), FRCS(Orth), FRCS(Eng), FRCS(Ed)
Foot and Ankle Unit, Royal Liverpool and Broadgreen University Hospitals, Liverpool, United Kingdom

BI-BO WANG, MD
Shanghai Ruijin Hospital, Shanghai Jiaotong University School of Medicine, Shanghai, China

MARTIN WEBER, MD
Professor, Department of Orthopaedic Surgery, Zieglerspital, University of Berne, Berne, Switzerland

WOLFRAM WENZ, MD
ATOS Clinic Heidelberg, Deutsches Gelenkzentrum Heidelberg, Heidelberg, Germany

XIANG-YANG XU, MD
Shanghai Ruijin Hospital, Shanghai Jiaotong University School of Medicine, Shanghai, China

YUAN ZHU, MD
Shanghai Ruijin Hospital, Shanghai Jiaotong University School of Medicine, Shanghai, China

Contents

William D. Harrison and Christopher R. Walker

> Current practices and controversies in bunion surgery in the United
> Kingdom are discussed in this article. Patients tend to be offered a distally
> based metatarsal osteotomy, such as a chevron or scarf osteotomy, for
> mild to moderate symptomatic bunions. Greater deformities are managed
> with a more extreme scarf, supplemented with a proximal phalangeal
> osteotomy. A proximal fusion in the form of the Lapidus-type procedure
> is still reserved for the most severe, hypermobile, or arthritic cases. Mini-
> mally invasive techniques for bunions have failed to disseminate into com-
> mon practice in the United Kingdom. The trends in the United Kingdom
> regarding litigation, venous thromboembolism, and osteodesis for bunion
> surgery are also discussed.

Sebastian Schmitt, Anna C. Peak, Gregor Berrsche, and Wolfram Wenz

> Foot deformities are found in several neurologic conditions; most typically,
> but not exclusively, Charcot-Marie-Tooth disease. Posttraumatic defor-
> mities and undercorrection, or overcorrection, of congenital talipes equi-
> novarus are also encountered. A severely deformed foot that cannot fit
> into normal shoes presents a significant day-to-day challenge to the young
> and active patient. This article presents some basic principles for evalu-
> ating the deformity and a toolkit of procedures to deal with these complex
> cases.

Yuan Zhu, Xiang-yang Xu, and Bi-bo Wang

> Foot and ankle physicians in China encounter quite a large amount of se-
> vere and complex deformities. The main cause of severe ankle and foot
> deformity is trauma, while the other causes may be neuromuscular dis-
> eases, improper reduction and fixation, and so on. Staged procedure
> may sometimes be a safer way to correct deformities in the presence of
> severe soft tissue contracture. Periarticular osteotomy combined with
> soft tissue balancing can be used in treating severe varus ankle arthritis,
> including stage IIIb cases and patients with talar tilt of more than 10
> degrees.

management. Obtaining good outcomes in these situations can be challenging. Often, the difference between average and good results has to
do with preoperative planning and good surgical technique. This article
outlines numerous techniques and tricks that are not always mentioned
in classic textbooks. It focuses on ankle, talus, calcaneus, and midfoot
fractures, and discusses numerous techniques and aids to avoid potential
problems that may be encountered intraoperatively.

The outcome after Lisfranc injuries correlates with anatomic and stable
reduction. The best surgical treatment, particularly for the ligamentous
Lisfranc injuries, remains controversial. Recent publications suggest
that the ligamentous injuries may benefit from primary partial Lisfranc
arthrodesis. Most surgeons agree that an appropriate reduction is better
and easier achieved by open reduction and stable temporary screw, by
dorsal plate fixation, by open primary partial arthrodesis than by closed
reduction, or by Kirschner wire fixation. Despite correct surgical technique and postoperative management, symptom-free recovery is uncommon. This article outlines current techniques in the management
of Lisfranc injuries and resultant postoperative outcomes in a level I
trauma center.

Study groups have been formed in France to advance the use of minimally
invasive surgery. These techniques are becoming more frequently used
and the technique nuances are continuing to evolve. The objective of
this article was to advance the awareness of the current trends in minimally
invasive surgery for common diseases of the forefoot. The percutaneous
surgery at the forefoot is less developed at this time, but will also be
discussed.

The ankle represents the most commonly injured weightbearing joint in the
human body. They are typically the result of low-energy, rotational injury
mechanisms. However, ankle fractures represent a spectrum of injury patterns from simple to very complex, with varying incidence of posttraumatic
arthritis. Stable injury patterns can be treated nonoperatively; unstable
injury patterns are typically treated operatively given that they could lead
to severe arthritis if not properly addressed.

Soccer is one of the most popular sports in the world. It has undergone
many changes in recent years, mainly because of increased physical demands, and this has led to an increased injury risk. Direct contact accounts

for half of all injuries in both indoor and outdoor soccer, and ankle sprains are the most common foot and ankle injury. There is a spectrum of foot and ankle injuries and their treatment should be individualized in these high-demand patients. An injury prevention program is also important and should be discussed between the players, the trainer, responsible physician, and physical therapists.

 Video content accompanies this article at http://www.foot.theclinics. com

Treatment of osteochondral defects (OCLs) of the talus is a challenging orthopedic surgery. Treatment of talar OCLs has evolved through the 3 "R" paradigm: reconstruction, repair, and replacement. This article highlights current state-of-the-art techniques and reviews recent advances in the literature about articular cartilage repair using various novel tissue engineering approaches, including various scaffolds, growth factors, and cell niches; which include chondrocytes and culture-expanded bone marrow-derived mesenchymal stem cells.

FOOT AND ANKLE CLINICS

RELATED INTEREST

Orthopedic Clinics of North America, April 2016 (Vol. 47, No. 2)
Common Complications in Orthopedics
James H. Calandruccio, Benjamin J. Grear, Benjamin M. Mauck,
Jeffrey R. Sawyer, Patrick C. Toy, and John C. Weinlein, *Editors*
Available at: www.emed.theclinics.com

THE CLINICS ARE NOW AVAILABLE ONLINE!
Access your subscription at:
www.theclinics.com

Preface

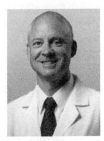 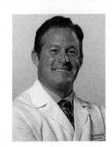

John G. Anderson, MD   Donald R. Bohay, MD, FACS
Editors

Today's world disseminates information at a rapid rate, with the Internet and social media bringing current events, in real time, into our homes. Progress occurs at a much faster pace than many of us are accustomed to. Innovation in health care is not only driven by technology, it is also driven by ideas. In this information age, the rapid spread of data allows all of us access to the same ideas and technology, regardless of nationality or location.

Internationally, the Foot and Ankle surgical specialty consists of a small network of individuals. *Foot and Ankle Clinics of North America* provides us with an excellent resource, which greatly improves our ability to bring leaders and innovative thinkers in our field together. This allows us all to share and learn from what is occurring around the world within our sphere. This issue of *Foot and Ankle Clinics of North America* seeks to highlight advancements and ideas that cross international borders. *Foot and Ankle Clinics of North America* does us all a great service by assembling this collaboration into a readily accessible and readable format that is available to those physicians who find it useful.

We are blessed to live in an era where surgeons in Turkey and Germany can openly and easily communicate with surgeons in Chile, Spain, England, and the United States to advance the science and knowledge of foot and ankle surgery. This issue represents a new age of global health care delivery, where access to modern technology is no longer limited by international boundaries. The cross-cultural reality of producing an article that has the potential to reach out to multiple audiences with different primary languages will not be lost on the reader. We can all learn from each other, and we are united in our goal to provide the best available foot and ankle orthopedic health care to our local and regional communities. The intention of this issue of *Foot and Ankle Clinics of North America* is to expand and enrich our communities.

There are many who deserve thanks for their assistance in putting this issue together. First and foremost, our appreciation goes out to all the authors, who have taken the time to allow us into their practice and to share their ideas. Second, our appreciation goes to the editorial staff at Elsevier, and to Mark Myerson, for their help at many stages of the process. Last, we would like to thank some individuals without whose help we would have run way past our deadline. This includes our

Foot Ankle Clin N Am 21 (2016) xiii–xiv
http://dx.doi.org/10.1016/j.fcl.2016.03.001
1083-7515/16/$ – see front matter © 2016 Published by Elsevier Inc.

foot.theclinics.com

fellows, Paul Butler, MD, Andrew Ertl, MD, Daniel Patton, MD, resident R. Stephen Otte, MD, and our research staff, Michelle A. Padley and Lindsey A. Behrend. This was a team effort, and we couldn't have completed this task without all of their efforts.

We truly hope you enjoy this issue of *Foot and Ankle Clinics of North America* as much as we have enjoyed putting it together.

John G. Anderson, MD
Orthopaedic Associates of Michigan
1111 Leffingwell Ave. Ne, Ste 100
Grand Rapids, MI 49525, USA

Donald R. Bohay, MD, FACS
Orthopaedic Associates of Michigan
1111 Leffingwell Ave. Ne, Ste 100
Grand Rapids, MI 49525, USA

E-mail addresses:
John.Anderson@oamichigan.com (J.G. Anderson)
Donald.Bohay@oamichigan.com (D.R. Bohay)

Controversies and Trends in United Kingdom Bunion Surgery

William D. Harrison, MBBS, MRCS, MSc,
Christopher R. Walker, MCh(Orth), FRCS(Orth), FRCS(Eng), FRCS(Ed)*

KEYWORDS

- Hallux valgus • Bunion • Surgery • Minimally invasive • Litigation

KEY POINTS

- The scarf metatarsal osteotomy is the most common surgery for bunions in the United Kingdom but it has a steep learning curve and can be used inappropriately.
- Controversy surrounds minimally invasive hallux valgus surgical techniques in the United Kingdom and they remain infrequently used because of a paucity of good evidence to support them at this stage.
- Litigation is declining but that could change following a recent judgment.
- Consensus on low venous thromboembolism risk in hallux valgus surgery is not matched by the national guidance that is currently issued.

INTRODUCTION

The earliest reports of surgery for bunions dates back to Gernet in 1836.[1] Over the last 180 years there have been many changes to the philosophy and techniques of hallux valgus management. In 1981, Helal[2] counted more than 150 described surgical techniques for hallux valgus correction, the inference being that there is no clear consensus on the best treatment of hallux valgus. A collective agreement has been made that those cases with mild to moderate hallux valgus, based on intermetatarsal angle (IMA) and hallux valgus angle (HVA), can be treated with a distally based translational osteotomy with or without rotation.[3]

Hallux valgus is a common problem, affecting an estimated 23% of adults aged 18–65 years and 35.7% more than 65 years of age based on international figures for an extensive epidemiologic literature review.[4] Hallux valgus management continues to be a topical discussion point in foot and ankle meetings in the United

Disclosure: The authors have nothing to disclose.
Foot and Ankle Unit, Royal Liverpool and Broadgreen University Hospitals, Prescot Street, Liverpool L7 8XP, UK
* Corresponding author.
E-mail address: Christopher.Walker@rlbuht.nhs.uk

Kingdom, and the greatest controversy still remains around minimally invasive surgery. The role of the Akin osteotomy, thromboembolic prophylaxis, and the effect of litigation on National Health Service (NHS) resources are also discussed.

CURRENT UNITED KINGDOM PRACTICE

Typical practice in the United Kingdom includes a chevron or short scarf osteotomy for mild hallux valgus,[5] and a scarf procedure performed for moderate disease. The technique for scarf osteotomy has developed over the last 10 years in the United Kingdom as a better understanding of the principles has been disseminated. Initially, practice varied considerably with a tendency to undertake the cut mainly in the diaphysis leading to guttering and shortening of the metatarsal. Concerns over transfer metatarsalgia led to an increased plantar sloping of the cut to offset the problem, which in turn reduced the true lateral translation and there was an overuse of the Akin procedure to overcome this.

Current practice promotes a cut positioned in the wider metaphyseal portions of the metatarsal in order to avoid the so-called gutter effect of diaphyseal overlap.[6] Greater confidence in prevention of guttering has resulted in a reduction in the plantar sloping of the cut, which allows greater scope for lateral displacement (**Fig. 1**). Although the scarf has been popular for IMAs of 14° to 18°,[7] it has tended to be used for greater and lesser angles, with or without an Akin procedure. It is becoming accepted that the greater the width of the metatarsal head, the greater the potential lateral displacement of the metatarsal osteotomy that is available before concerns about instability arise. Therefore, algorithms based purely on IMA are modified, extending the potential of a translational osteotomy.

More severe deformities, with an IMA greater than 18°, can be treated with a proximal metatarsal osteotomy or fusion of either the first metatarsophalangeal joint or the first tarsometatarsal joint. In the United Kingdom, there is a trend away from performing basal metatarsal osteotomies for severe hallux valgus. First, when the distal metatarsal articular angle is increased preoperatively, especially in younger patients, they are likely to be left with greater incongruence.[8] Second, recurrence in these larger deformities is common, probably because of the inherent instability of the first tarsometatarsal joint, which contributes significantly to the deformity in the first place (**Figs. 2 and 3**).

In UK practice, severe hallux valgus, especially in the presence of first tarsometatarsal osteoarthritis or hypermobility, is now more commonly treated with a Lapidus-type procedure, usually undertaken using a variety of fixation techniques, which is different from those popularized by Lapidus in 1960 and Hansen[9] in 1996. The advent of locking

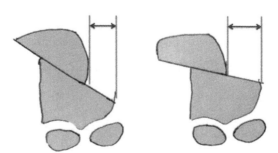

Fig. 1. Increased translation is possible for a given percentage width with a decrease in the slope of the scarf cut.

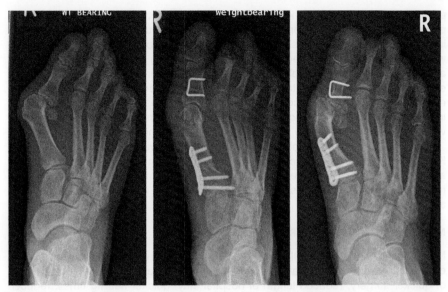

Fig. 2. Recurrence of first metatarsal varus following a basal osteotomy in a patient with a preoperative severe IMA.

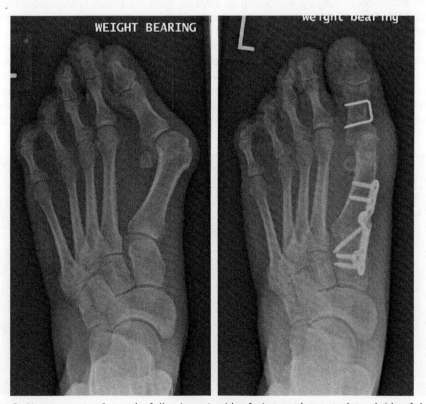

Fig. 3. Nonrecurrence 6 months following a Lapidus fusion on the contralateral side of the same patient.

plates has contributed to the increasing confidence of UK surgeons to undertake this procedure. This increased confidence has been backed up by cadaver[10,11] and clinical studies.[12] A Swiss study showed the importance of good compression at the joint with an interfragmentary screw in addition to the locking plate to achieve stability,[13] and the high incidence of metalwork removal (17%)[12] remains a concern. Improved evidence is required to ascertain whether the additional cost of these devices is warranted compared with less costly screw-only techniques. However, if the theoretic improved fixation translates to clinically improved outcomes with earlier mobilization, weight bearing, and return to work, then it is likely that these will be cost-effective.

Very-low-demand elderly patients with severe hallux valgus may still be offered a Keller procedure in the United Kingdom, especially when they are home ambulators and not capable of protective weight bearing. It also remains useful in the management of ulcerated bunions, especially in the presence of increased patient morbidity and diabetes (**Fig. 4**).

MINIMALLY INVASIVE SURGERY

Minimally invasive surgery (MIS) has gained popularity in all fields of surgery. In general, the philosophy of minimal soft tissue disruption comes with the potential benefits of quicker surgery, reduced length of hospital stay, quicker healing times, reduced pain scores, and smaller scars.

MIS for hallux valgus can include percutaneous surgery, minimal incision surgery, and arthroscopic surgery. According to advisers from the British Orthopaedic Foot and Ankle Society, it is estimated that less than 10% of UK foot and ankle surgeons perform MIS bunion surgery at present.

The National Institute for Health and Care Excellence (NICE) has issued recommendations for MIS for hallux valgus in the United Kingdom (NICE IPG332, issued February 2010). The theoretic concerns of MIS (as stated by the advisers to NICE) include burning soft tissue, tendon injury, disruption to local blood supply, inflammatory reaction to bone debris, first metatarsal malpositioning, shortening, or avascular necrosis. Many of these complications are in direct contrast with the theoretic advantages of

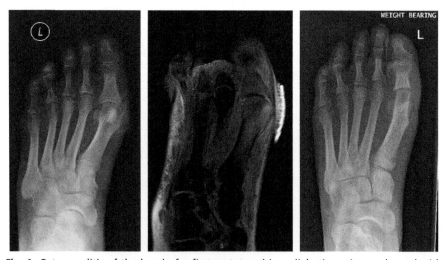

Fig. 4. Osteomyelitis of the head of a first metatarsal in a diabetic patient, salvaged with intravenous antibiotic therapy and a Keller procedure.

MIS surgery as stated earlier. The NICE committee recommends that clinicians performing minimally invasive bunion surgery in the United Kingdom conduct a local audit of outcomes.

Percutaneous distal osteotomies were an emerging technique from both Europe and the United States during the 1990s, and were used for mild to moderate hallux valgus.[14,15] Several techniques have been described, including the Bösch method[14] and the Reverdin technique, modified by Isham[15] in 1991; the Simple Effective Reliable and Inexpensive (SERI) osteotomy[16] and; also the minimally invasive chevron-Akin (MICA).[17]

The Reverdin-Isham technique used a modified Shannon burr to perform an oblique medial closing wedge osteotomy of the head of the first metatarsal along with a bunionectomy, adductor release, and a minimally invasive Akin procedure.[17] There was no routine internal fixation used and the mean shortening of the first metatarsal was 5 mm. A dynamic plantar pressure distribution study of 20 feet that had undergone the Reverdin-Isham technique showed an increase in pressure to the lesser metatarsal heads and no meaningful change to the pressure exerted to the first metatarsal head.[18] Despite the lack of fixation and metatarsal shortening, Isham[15] published long-term clinical outcomes with good results. Bauer and colleagues,[19,20] an independent group using the Reverdin-Isham osteotomy, described a sharp learning curve and limited the indications to mild-moderate hallux valgus. At 2 years' follow-up, their results from 104 cases were comparable with, but no better than, existing percutaneous techniques.[19,20]

The Bösch technique is currently the most commonly performed minimally invasive method across Europe and uses a percutaneous subcapital osteotomy under fluoroscopic guidance and a high-speed power burr. The associated complications are similar to the Reverdin-Isham technique but, in addition, a percutaneous K wire is used as stabilization for 6 weeks with associated stiffness in 31% and pin-site infection of 0.9% to 15%.[21–23]

A small-scale randomized controlled trial by Giannini and colleagues[16] compared SERI, a monoplanar shortening distal metatarsal osteotomy, with a traditional rigid screw fixation of a scarf osteotomy. Twenty patients with bilateral hallux valgus were randomly assigned either SERI or scarf procedures to each foot. There were no differences reported between the groups other than reduced time in theater for the SERI osteotomy. Stiffness and reduced motion were reported in 15% of both comparative procedures. The groups had similar radiographic outcomes and similar improvements in American Orthopaedic Foot and Ankle Society (AOFAS) scores.[16] Although Giannini and colleagues[16] found the SERI to be favorable, a prospective study by Kadakia and colleagues[24] described universally poor outcomes for the SERI osteotomy, with complications including union (70%), recurrence (40%), osteonecrosis, and wound complications.[17] The additional outcomes of shortening and stiffening are not considered acceptable in UK practice and therefore are not performed.

The newest addition to the percutaneous techniques, called MICA, comes from Vernois and Redfern, who use a chevron-type osteotomy at the level of the distal diaphyseal-metaphyseal junction of the first metatarsal and an Akin-type phalangeal osteotomy with percutaneous soft tissue releases. Both osteotomies are internally fixed with compression screws.[17] The results from 83 cases with 12-month follow-up have satisfactory HVA and IMA correction, 7% malunion, 5% transfer metatarsalgia, 1.5% superficial wound infections, no cases of osteonecrosis, and an overall 94% patient satisfaction rate.[17] This technique seems to hold the greatest chance of longer-term success. However, the learning curve is long and although Vernois and

Redfern continue to popularize the technique, several UK surgeons have moved back to open surgery for their metatarsal osteotomies, although there is increasing evidence for the effectiveness of the cheilectomy and Akin using this less invasive procedure.[17,25]

Arthroscopic surgery for hallux valgus has also been described as a means to achieve a lateral soft tissue release and guide screw placement. It is not generally used in the United Kingdom. A cadaveric study of arthroscopic lateral soft tissue release showed no incidence of neural or cartilage damage. A clinical study with level IV evidence from the same unit reported 94 cases undergoing arthroscopic surgery with a postoperative AOFAS pain score of 37 out of 40 and a 95.7% patient satisfaction rate.[26] Complications included recurrence (2.1%), hallux varus (1.1%), screw breakage (1.1%), skin-knot impingement (1.1%), and revision (3%).

The largest review article of minimally invasive bunion surgery, by Trnka and colleagues,[1] appeared in 2013. They identified 21 articles describing the results from 1750 patients undergoing 2195 surgeries. Of these articles, 1 was level II evidence,[16] 3 were level III evidence,[22,23,27] and the rest were level IV evidence. Most of the articles were reported by advocates of the technique. The review concluded that the stated complications were under-reported, compared with their own experience in clinical practice.[1] The overall conclusion from this review article was that there is a paucity of high-level evidence regarding MIS for hallux valgus. This finding correlates with the same conclusions from the NICE select committee in the United Kingdom.

According to 3 studies, the reported postoperative improvements to the HVA following all types of MIS for bunion surgery are 26° to 7.5° ($P<.01$),[28] 33° to 14° ($P<.05$),[26] and 32° to 14.1° ($P = .04$).[29] The changes in HVA are comparable with those seen with traditional scarf osteotomies, with a mean change of 34.6° to 14.9° in one series.[30] Patients with an HVA greater than 30° have poor results following percutaneous bunion surgery. Huang and colleagues[31] showed that 64% (23 out of 36 patients) had a poor radiological result, defined as a postoperative HVA of 20° or more.

Some complications from MIS bunion surgery are similar to those of open surgery, such as chronic regional pain syndrome at between 2% and 6%.[20,22] However, nonunion (5.5%–10%)[22,32] and osteonecrosis seem to be higher. Osteonecrosis has been reported as 4.2% in a series of 72 cases.[32] Tendon injury has also been anecdotally reported but not substantiated in the literature.

There is a growing demand for MIS bunion surgery from patients in the United Kingdom. This demand comes as a result of newspaper and magazine articles, despite the lack of medium-term studies on MIS procedures. There is a potentially a large impact on the NHS if the practice in the private sector translates into mainstream UK practice. As such, there is a need for a large-scale randomized-controlled trial to draw conclusions about the short-term and long-term results. Given the rapid uptake of the scarf osteotomy in the United Kingdom during the 1990s, it is likely that MIS could follow a similar trend if proved to be superior for mild to moderate hallux valgus.

AKIN PROCEDURE

Controversy remains about the need to perform an Akin osteotomy. Originally described by Akin in 1925, this is now the common term used for a medial closing wedge periarticular angulation osteotomy of the hallux proximal phalanx. It primarily works best for hallux valgus interphalangeus. However, it is used more often as a supplement to inadequate correction of the intermetatarsal angle during hallux valgus surgery. In general, there should not be an over-reliance on the Akin procedure to correct an excessive residual hallux valgus following the metatarsal osteotomy. This deformity should be corrected by the metatarsal osteotomy or more proximal fusion. Improvement of surgical technique to achieve greater translation of the metatarsal head or moving to a more proximal realignment technique is required. A large Akin osteotomy in the presence of an undercorrected metatarsal osteotomy leads to an S-shaped first ray (**Figs. 5** and **6**).

NOVEL FIXATION TECHNIQUES

Modern financial and political pressures on the NHS in the United Kingdom have led to the development of suture fixation techniques to reduce the cost of hallux valgus surgery. Suture fixation for the Akin procedure was shown by Cullen and colleagues[33] to be cost-effective and to have a 0% malunion and nonunion rate in a series of 115 cases. Despite this, many UK surgeons continue to worry about the strength of fixation following this technique, requiring a return to theater, and therefore making it not at all cost-effective. The biomechanical strength of suture fixation of Akin osteotomies has not been tested. The most rigid Akin fixation constructs were crossed K wires when compared with 4 other internal fixation devices, such as 2-hole plates and interfragmentary screws.[34] Despite this study, the prominence of wires makes this an unusual fixation device for this procedure in the United Kingdom. The commonest fixation technique is an oblique dual-threaded headless screw.

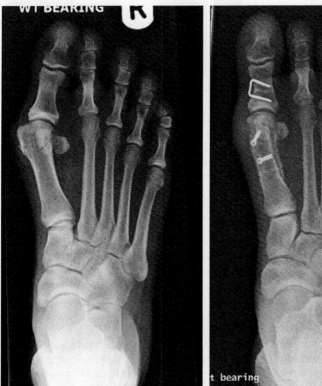
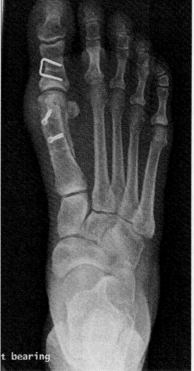

Fig. 5. Inadequate translation of a scarf osteotomy with an uncovered sesamoid improved with an Akin osteotomy but leaving the patient with a wide foot.

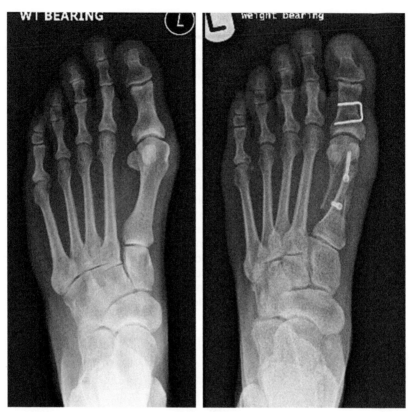

Fig. 6. Satisfactory translation with covered sesamoids and an additional Akin procedure to correct an 8° interphalangeus deformity.

Suture-based osteodesis devices have been developed that reduce the IMA between the first and second metatarsals. They are not commonly used in the United Kingdom. This finding is supported by several studies showing high rates of complications, including hardware failure (5.6%), hallux varus (3.6%), joint subluxations (4%), and stress fractures (5%–31%).[35–37]

VENOUS THROMBOEMBOLIC PROPHYLAXIS

Evidence from reported data in United Kingdom from 33,626 patients undergoing first metatarsal osteotomies shows a deep vein thrombosis rate of 0.01%, pulmonary embolism rate of 0.02%, and a mortality of 0.04%.[38] The article showed no clear risk factors for venous thromboembolism (VTE) events in bunion surgery and VTE prophylaxis had no evidence of benefit in these ambulatory cases. Regardless of the evidence, prophylaxis is generally given to those who have a further risk factor for VTE, such as a nonambulatory status, history of previous VTE, prolonged surgery (>90 minutes), and multiple medical comorbidities. Practice tends to vary around the United Kingdom; however, NICE guidelines considers all patients undergoing inpatient orthopedic lower limb surgery lasting more than 90 minutes to be at increased risk and recommend chemical and mechanical VTE prophylaxis. Patients who are ambulatory after day case surgery are not considered at high risk of VTE. UK foot and ankle surgeons seem to have good consensus regarding assessing all patients for risk factors and reasonable consensus that uncomplicated forefoot surgery should be considered low risk. However, this does not correlate with the NICE guidance because the foot is part of the lower limb. This situation results in overtreatment of patients who are kept in overnight, because most accept chemical prophylaxis if offered. It is now 5 years since the release of the guidance and attempts are continuing to influence the next update to provide more appropriate advice for forefoot patients.

LITIGATION

Foot and ankle surgery accounted for 12.6% (N = 1294) of 10,273 orthopedic litigation claims in England and Wales over a 17-year period.[39] This review of NHS litigation data from Ring and colleagues[39] showed that overall frequency of litigation is low in UK first-ray procedures at 2.26% (N = 232). However, this was the second most common area for litigation in the foot and ankle and the most common for elective practice.[39] Claims were most frequently made for incorrect selection or poorly performed procedures for hallux valgus.

There was a steady increase in trauma and orthopedic litigation in England and Wales reported to the NHS Litigation Authority (NHSLA) from 1995, plateauing in the early 2000s.[40] This increase has been reflected in the foot and ankle subgroup. There was a development of more stringent guidelines by the General Medical Council (GMC) on consent in 2008, which coincides with an increase in numbers from 2008 to 2009. An improved patient consent process has been encouraged since then and this has coincided with a decrease in litigation numbers, including in foot and ankle procedures.[39] The authors' preferred method is to consent the patient in a dedicated preoperative clinic, dictating the dialogue and relevant risks in the clinic letter, copying to the patient, and supported by patient information leaflets. Consenting the patient in an outpatient environment seems to significantly reduce the risk of litigation.[41] The NHSLA figures discussed earlier could change again in the next few years following a recent Supreme Court ruling that enshrines the GMC 2008 guidance in law. The ruling has brought in a new test on information used to inform a patient of risks of a procedure: "The test of materiality is whether, in the circumstances of the particular case, a reasonable person in the patient's position would be likely to attach significance to the risk, or the doctor is or should reasonably be aware that the particular patient would be likely to attach significance to it." This is a move away from the concept of the reasonable doctor (Bolam test) to the reasonable patient.[42] (Further guidance is available from the Medical Protection Society.)

In a difficult economic environment, improved patient involvement in decisions on treatment and accurate record keeping are becoming essential in the United Kingdom. This improvement seems to be reducing the number of claims, which may reflect more realistic expectations from patients.

REFERENCES

1. Trnka H-J, Krenn S, Schuh R. Minimally invasive hallux valgus surgery: a critical review of the evidence. Int Orthop 2013;37(9):1731–5.
2. Helal B. Surgery for adolescent hallux valgus. Clin Orthop Relat Res 1981;(157): 50–63.
3. Trnka HJ, Zembsch A, Easley ME, et al. The chevron osteotomy for correction of hallux valgus. Comparison of findings after two and five years of follow-up. J Bone Joint Surg Am 2000;82-A:1373–8.
4. Nix S, Smith M, Vicenzino B. Prevalence of hallux valgus in the general population: a systematic review and meta-analysis. J Foot Ankle Res 2010;3:21.

5. Weil LS. Scarf osteotomy for correction of hallux valgus. Historical perspective, surgical technique, and results. Foot Ankle Clin 2000;5(3):559–80.

6. Coetzee JC. Scarf osteotomy for hallux valgus repair: the dark side. Foot Ankle Int 2003;24(1):29–33.

7. Kristen KH, Berger C, Stelzig S, et al. The SCARF osteotomy for the correction of hallux valgus deformities. Foot Ankle Int 2002;23(3):221–9.

8. Robinson AHN, Limbers JP. Modern concepts in the treatment of hallux valgus. J Bone Joint Surg Br 2005;87:1038–45.

9. Hansen ST. Hallux valgus surgery. Morton and Lapidus were right! Clin Podiatr Med Surg 1996;13(3):347–54.

10. Scranton PE, Coetzee JC, Carreira D. Arthrodesis of the first metatarsocuneiform joint: a comparative study of fixation methods. Foot Ankle Int 2009;30(4):341–5.

11. Cottom JM, Rigby RB. Biomechanical comparison of a locking plate with intra-plate compression screw versus locking plate with plantar interfragmentary screw for Lapidus arthrodesis: a cadaveric study. J Foot Ankle Surg 2013; 52(3):339–42.

12. Cottom JM, Vora AM. Fixation of Lapidus arthrodesis with a plantar interfragmentary screw and medial locking plate: a report of 88 cases. J Foot Ankle Surg 2013; 52(4):465–9.

13. Klos K, Gueorguiev B, Mückley T, et al. Stability of medial locking plate and compression screw versus two crossed screws for Lapidus arthrodesis. Foot Ankle Int 2010;31(2):158–63.

14. Bosch P, Wanke S, Legenstein R. Hallux valgus correction by the method of Bosch: a new technique with a seven-to-ten-year follow-up. Foot Ankle Clin 2000;5(3):485–98, v–vi.

15. Isham SA. The Reverdin-Isham procedure for the correction of hallux abducto valgus. A distal metatarsal osteotomy procedure. Clin Podiatr Med Surg 1991; 8(1):81–94.

16. Giannini S, Cavallo M, Faldini C, et al. The SERI distal metatarsal osteotomy and scarf osteotomy provide similar correction of hallux valgus. Clin Orthop Relat Res 2013;471(7):2305–11.

17. Redfern D, Perera AM. Minimally invasive osteotomies. Foot Ankle Clin 2014; 19(2):181–9.

18. Rodríguez-Reyes G, López-Gavito E, Pérez-Sanpablo AI, et al. Dynamic plantar pressure distribution after percutaneous hallux valgus correction using the Reverdin-Isham osteotomy. Rev Invest Clin 2014;66(Suppl 1):S79–84.

19. Bauer T, de Lavigne C, Biau D, et al. Percutaneous hallux valgus surgery: a prospective multicenter study of 189 cases. Orthop Clin North Am 2009;40(4): 505–14, ix.

20. Bauer T, Biau D, Lortat-Jacob A. Percutaneous hallux valgus correction using the Reverdin-Isham osteotomy. Orthop Traumatol Surg Res 2010;96(4):407–16.

21. Markowski HP, Bosch P, Rannicher V. Surgical technique and preliminary results of a percutaneous neck osteotomy of the first metatarsal for hallux valgus. Foot 1991;2(2):93–8.

22. Roth A, Kohlmaier W, Tschauner C. Surgery of hallux valgus. Distal metatarsal osteotomy—subcutaneous ("Bösch") versus open ("Kramer") procedures. Foot Ankle Surg 1996;2(2):109–17.

23. Maffulli N, Longo UG, Oliva F, et al. Bosch osteotomy and scarf osteotomy for hallux valgus correction. Orthop Clin North Am 2009;40(4):515–24.

24. Kadakia AR, Smerek JP, Myerson MS. Radiographic results after percutaneous distal metatarsal osteotomy for correction of hallux valgus deformity. Foot Ankle Int 2007;28(3):355–60.

25. Redfern D, Vernois J, Legré BP. Percutaneous surgery of the forefoot. Clin Podiatr Med Surg 2015;32(3):291–332.

26. Lui TH, Chan KB, Chow HT, et al. Arthroscopy-assisted correction of hallux valgus deformity. Arthroscopy 2008;24(8):875–80.

27. Radwan YA, Mansour AM. Percutaneous distal metatarsal osteotomy versus distal chevron osteotomy for correction of mild-to-moderate hallux valgus deformity. Arch Orthop Trauma Surg 2012;132(11):1539–46.

28. Weinberger BH, Fulp JM, Falstrom P, et al. Retrospective evaluation of percutaneous bunionectomies and distal osteotomies without internal fixation. Clin Podiatr Med Surg 1991;8(1):111–36.

29. Maffulli N, Oliva F, Coppola C, et al. Minimally invasive hallux valgus correction: a technical note and a feasibility study. J Surg Orthop Adv 2005;14(4):193–8.

30. Adam SP, Choung SC, Gu Y, et al. Outcomes after scarf osteotomy for treatment of adult hallux valgus deformity. Clin Orthop Relat Res 2011;469(3):854–9.

31. Huang PJ, Lin YC, Fu YC, et al. Radiographic evaluation of minimally invasive distal metatarsal osteotomy for hallux valgus. Foot Ankle Int 2011;32(5):S503–7.

32. Iannò B, Familiari F, De Gori M, et al. Midterm results and complications after minimally invasive distal metatarsal osteotomy for treatment of hallux valgus. Foot Ankle Int 2013;34(7):969–77.

33. Cullen NP, Angel J, Singh D, et al. Fixation of an akin osteotomy with a tension suture: our results. Foot (Edinb) 2009;19:107–9.

34. Chacon Y, Fallat LM, Dau N, et al. Biomechanical comparison of internal fixation techniques for the Akin osteotomy of the proximal phalanx. J Foot Ankle Surg 2012;51(5):561–5.

35. Dayton P, Sedberry S, Feilmeier M. Complications of metatarsal suture techniques for bunion correction: a systematic review of the literature. J Foot Ankle Surg 2015;54(2):230–2.

36. Weatherall JM, Chapman CB, Shapiro SL. Postoperative second metatarsal fractures associated with suture-button implant in hallux valgus surgery. Foot Ankle Int 2013;34(1):104–10.

37. Wu DY, Lam KF. Osteodesis for hallux valgus correction: is it effective? Clin Orthop Relat Res 2014;473(1):328–36.

38. Jameson SS, Augustine A, James P, et al. Venous thromboembolic events following foot and ankle surgery in the English National Health Service. J Bone Joint Surg Br 2011;93(4):490–7.

39. Ring J, Talbot CL, Clough TM. Clinical negligence in foot and ankle surgery: a 17-year review of claims to the NHS Litigation Authority. Bone Joint J 2014;96-B(11):1510–4.

40. Atrey A, Gupte CM, Corbett SA. Review of successful litigation against English health trusts in the treatment of adults with orthopaedic pathology: clinical governance lessons learned. J Bone Joint Surg Am 2010;92(18):e36.

41. Bhattacharyya T, Yeon H, Harris MB. The medical-legal aspects of informed consent in orthopaedic surgery. J Bone Joint Surg 2005;87(11):2395–400.

42. Reid E. Montgomery v Lanarkshire Health Board and the rights of the reasonable patient. Edinburgh Law Review 2015;19(3):360–6.

What's New in Severe Deformity Correction
The German Perspective

Sebastian Schmitt, MD[a],*, Anna C. Peak, FRCS (Orth)[b],
Gregor Berrsche, MD[a], Wolfram Wenz, MD[a]

KEYWORDS

- Osteotomy • Foot deformities • Fusion • Chopart joint • Tendon transfer
- Arthrodesis

KEY POINTS

- Bone biology is more important than absolute stability and compression.
- The goal of treatment is a pain-free, plantigrade, shoeable foot; this is more important than joint preservation.
- In neurogenic deformity, fusions reduce recurrence rates.
- The bony correction should take place around the center of rotation angle of the deformity, which in most cases is at the Chopart joint.
- Tendon transfers and soft tissue correction alone cannot correct deformity. However, tendon transfers are essential in addition to fusions to balance the foot.

INTRODUCTION: NATURE OF THE PROBLEM

Hindfoot and midfoot deformities can occur secondary to several neurologic and congenital conditions, and neurologic conditions can cause different foot deformities. However, a variety of deformities can be approached using the same broad treatment principles.

This article outlines these principles and then discusses some example cases. This approach is suitable in cases of Charcot-Marie-Tooth disease, cerebral palsy, spina bifida, clubfoot, and polio. However, the management of Charcot arthropathy is not discussed because this requires a different approach.

INDICATIONS

Every severe foot deformity, such as cavus foot, cavovarus foot, calcaneal foot, equinus foot, and equinocavovarus foot.

Disclosure: The authors have nothing to disclose.
[a] ATOS Clinic Heidelberg, Deutsches Gelenkzentrum Heidelberg, Bismarckstraße 9 - 15, Heidelberg 69115, Germany; [b] Heatherwood and Wexham Park Hospitals, Ascot, UK
* Correspondence:
E-mail address: Sebastian.schmitt1810@gmail.com

CONTRAINDICATIONS

- Vascular disease of the lower limb
- High-grade infection
- Osteomyelitis

SURGICAL TECHNIQUE/PROCEDURE

The aim of surgery is to achieve a pain-free, plantigrade, shoeable foot. Patients should be prepared to consent to personalized correction, including bone graft. The exact operative plan may need to be modified intraoperatively.

The procedures can be divided into basic 4 steps undertaken in this order:

1. Release/harvest of the tendons needed for tendon transfers and sometimes the Achilles tendon
2. Bony correction of the hindfoot
3. Bony correction of the forefoot to fit the repositioned hindfoot
4. Tensioning and fixation of the transferred tendons

The bony correction starts with the fusion of the talonavicular joint.

The authors prefer to use Kirschner (K) wires for fixation, especially in younger patients, because this leaves a greater surface area of healing bone to unite the fusion site. Either 2 or 3 wires are used across the fusion site and are left in for 6 weeks before being removed in the plaster room. In addition, the authors frequently temporarily transfix the ankle joint in a neutral position for 2 to 6 weeks. This method allows for easy tensioning and protection of the tendon transfers and avoids plaster errors in the postoperative period.

Hindfoot/Midfoot Procedures

- Chopart fusion (Imhäuser procedure)
- Triple fusion
- Triple fusion with Lambrinudi procedure
- All of the above can be augmented by corrective osteotomies; for example, lateral closed Dwyer osteotomy

Forefoot Procedures

- First metatarsal dorsiflexion osteotomy, Tubby procedure
- Modified Jones procedure for claw hallux
- Russel-Hibbs procedure for claw toes

Soft Tissue Correction

- Total split posterior tibial tendon transfer (T-SPOTT) to the tibialis anterior and peroneus brevis tendon
- Steindler procedure to transect the plantar aponeurosis
- Achilles/gastrocnemius tendon lengthening (distal or proximal)

PREOPERATIVE PLANNING

The planning must include the full history, including any previous treatment and diagnoses, especially the type of neurogenic or spastic disease.

In cases of childhood deformity and unclear primary disease, the history should include precise details of complications during pregnancy and childbirth. Furthermore, the growth of the child should be assessed.

Observation of the Patient

- From the back of the patient: heel elevation, varus/valgus deformity of the heel, pronation of forefoot with too-many-toes sign, supination of the forefoot with hello-big-toe sign, rotational profile of the ankle
- Lateral view: lengthened/shortened foot arch, flattened/prominent lateral border, prominent fifth metatarsal base, prominent talar head on the dorsum of the foot, rotational profile of the ankle, ulceration at the lateral border, callosities
- Medial view: elevated/flattened heel, increased/flattened medial arch, elevated/decreased first metatarsal head, rotation of the malleolus, position of the talar head
- From the front of the patient: position of the talar head, rotation of the malleolus, prominence of the lateral/medial foot border, forefoot supination/pronation, forefoot adduction/abduction, clawing toes, diagonal skin folds
- Plantar view: foot shape, position of the fifth metatarsal, adduction/abduction of the forefoot, increased weight bearing on the metatarsal heads with increased callosities, weight bearing of the heel, ulceration of the skin

EXAMINATION

- The stiffness of the deformity of the hindfoot-, midfoot, and forefoot to reach a passive plantigrade foot arch is significant for the therapy.
- The range of motion of the ankle, particularly dorsiflexion, is to be assessed with focus on the bony impingement of the talus to the distal tibia. The examination is performed with the knee flexed and straight.
- The stiffness of the plantar aponeurosis and the intrinsic muscles has to be assessed in the cavus foot. The manual examination of the talonavicular joint is important to assess the grade of the medial subluxation of the navicular bone or the talar head and the stiffness of the joint subluxation, which can be tested with passive mobilization in abduction eversion direction. In addition, subluxation of the cuboid has to be assessed. While testing the mobility of these joints, the examiner can assess the passive correction of the midfoot and forefoot. The stiffness of the subtalar joint should be assessed.
- The muscular activity of the tibialis anterior/posterior, peronei, and flexor/extensor hallucis/digitorum has to be assessed. A muscular weakness or overload should be documented.
- The active/passive mobility of the toes allows an assessment of the intrinsic and extrinsic muscles.

COLEMAN BLOCK TEST

The Coleman Block Test is used to distinguish a fixed hindfoot varus and a flexible hindfoot varus by balancing the upright first metatarsus.[1] The hindfoot is underlaid by a block. By taking any fixed pronation of the forefoot out of play, the flexible hindfoot varus can correct. In the case of fixed hindfoot varus, there is no hindfoot correction.

SILFVERSKIÖLD TEST

The Silfverskiöld Test is used to distinguish between tension of the gastrocnemius and soleus muscle. Dorsiflexion is measured with the knee bent, then the hip and knee joint are extended slowly. While extending the knee, the gastrocnemius is tensioned. A significant difference in dorsiflexion of the foot while bending and extending the knee shows a gastrocnemius component on the equinus foot. If there is no difference in the dorsiflexion of the foot, the soleus muscle is also tight.

DYNAMIC EXAMINATION

- Examination of the stance and gait phases should be done
- Examination of the heel contact
- Limited dorsiflexion with reduced roll-off ability
- Examination of the first contact of the toes
- Compensatory hyperextension or flexion contracture of the knees
- Fixed flexion of the hips during stance and gait phases
- Foot progression angle
- Proximal examination of the spine
- Photography and video recording of the patient is always recommended for the treating surgeon and the patient to document progress

ADDITIONS

In addition to the dynamic and clinical examination, dynamic pedobarography is an effective method to measure the pressure distribution pattern. The measurement shows the major locations of pressure of the foot caused by the deformity.

RADIOGRAPHIC ASSESSMENT

- Weight-bearing anteroposterior (AP) and lateral radiographs of the feet and of the ankles are essential.
- Three-dimensional imaging is not routinely used in the preoperative planning stage, but can be useful in the postoperative phase, especially computed tomography scan, if there are concerns as to the union of an arthrodesis.
- The joints should be assessed for degenerative disease.
- In the AP foot radiograph, the main focus is the talonavicular joint. In cases of cavus deformity, the talonavicular joint is subluxed with medial subluxation of the navicular bone. The talus takes a position parallel to the calcaneus with radiological overlaying to each other. In addition, the fifth metatarsal is radiologically overlaid by the medial metatarsals with adduction of the first metatarsal relative to the talar head. Furthermore, the calcaneocuboid joint is subluxed with medial subluxation of the cuboid bone. In a planus deformity, the forefoot is supinated and abducted. In this case, the navicular is mostly shaped like a triangle with an additional external tibial bone.
- In the lateral foot radiograph, in which there is a cavus component to the deformity, the longitudinal calcaneal axis and the longitudinal talar axis are parallel to each other. The fibula is externally rotated. A calcaneal varus position is accompanied by a sinus tarsi window. The cuboid bone is not radiologically overlaid by the navicular bone. There is a prominent fifth metatarsal on the plantar side. The base of the first metatarsal is elevated. In the case of planus component, the cuboid cannot be separated in the lateral view from the navicular bone. The naviculocuneiform joint is depressed. The metatarsals are overlaid. The height of the foot arch is reduced. No sinus tarsi window is seen. Talar beaking by the navicular bone may be seen. In addition, the examiner should assess a ventral or dorsal impingement of the talus.
- In the AP radiograph of the ankle, the examiner is able to assess the varus or valgus position of the talar head in the tibiotalar joint and the position of the medial and lateral malleolus.

PREOPERATIVE PLANNING

The preoperative planning includes the clinical and dynamic examination, the radiographs, and the dynamic pedobarography. Nevertheless, the clinical examination should be repeated under anesthesia before beginning surgical treatment.

PATIENT POSITIONING

The authors prefer the supine position on the operating table. Every patient should consent to autologous bone graft from the iliac crest. Therefore, the authors always drape the iliac crest into the operative field. The authors normally use a thigh tourniquet. A sterile draped pillow under the calf muscles is used to lift the foot, if needed.

SURGICAL APPROACH

- The authors prefer different surgical approaches in surgical correction of foot deformities.
- The medial skin incision above the origin of the plantar aponeurosis is used for the Steindler procedure.
- The medial incision on the medial back side of the foot is used for Chopart; triple arthrodesis, including Lambrinudi procedure; Cole procedure; and the tibial tendon transfer.
- The lateral incision on the lateral back side of the foot is also used for the Chopart; triple arthrodesis, including Lambrinudi procedure; Cole procedure; and the tibial tendon transfer.
- A medial distal shank incision is used for lengthening of the Achilles tendon.
- The ventral shank incision of the tibia is needed for the tibial anterior/posterior/ flexor hallucis/flexor digitorum transfer.
- The dorsal S-shaped incision on the first metatarsal is used for the modified Jones procedure.

SURGICAL PROCEDURES
Bony Correction

Chopart (Imhäuser) or triple fusion
Indication
  The indication for Chopart and triple fusion is a rigid fixed adducted or supinated forefoot in deformity without varus hindfoot.[2–5]

Procedure
- Performing the fusion of the Chopart joint line, the authors use lateral and medial incisions to have the best overview of both joints and to secure the complete removal of the cartilage.
- The medial incision is made arch shaped in the length of 3 to 4 cm 1 finger distally of the medial malleolus to the navicular. Incise the subcutaneous tissue, the flexor retinaculum, and the sheath of the tibialis posterior tendon. Mobilize the tendon carefully with a chisel for retraction or release it with a scalpel on the border to the navicular for later tendon transfer. Insert 2 Vierstein retractors in the same way as on the lateral side to expose the talonavicular joint while incising and resecting the joint capsule.
- The lateral arch-shaped skin incision begins 2 cm distally to the lateral malleolus and ends distally to the talar head. Expose the sural and cutaneus dorsalis intermedius nerves and vessels and secure and mark these with a vessel loop while

retracting these in a proximal direction. After exposing the extensor digitorum brevis and peroneus brevis tendons, release the extensor digitorum brevis tendon with an L-shaped incision to get access to the Chopart joint line. Use a second vessel loop to mark the tendon. After insertion of 2 Vierstein retractors under the medial and lateral wound border, the Chopart joint line can be opened with incision and resection of the capsule.

- Reduce the foot manually, centering the navicular on the talar head. If the reduction is satisfactory and a plantigrade foot shape is achieved, the next step is the removal of the cartilage with a chisel. If the reduction and correction of the adducted forefoot are unsatisfactory, use an oscillating saw to resect a dorsally based wedge-shaped slice 0.5 cm thick from the Chopart joint to avoid overcorrection. The cancellous parts of the bony resection should be collected for eventual bony defect filling.
- Penetrate the subchondral bone with a chisel or a drill to promote the bony fusion. Set the foot to the plantigrade axis. Use 2.5-mm to 3.0-mm K wires to stabilize the reduced joints. The authors prefer to take 2 2K wires for the talonavicular and 2 for the calcaneocuboid joint. The authors prefer retrograde drilling of the K wires. Check the wire position with intraoperative radiographs.
- In cases of unsatisfactory correction of the foot after Chopart joint line resection by virtue of a severe hindfoot varus, the arthrodesis has to be extended to the subtalar joint (triple arthrodesis). Remove all fatty and fibrous tissue from the sinus tarsi. Retract the peroneal tendons with a Vierstein retractor. Open the joint capsule. Remove the cartilage of the ventral and dorsal compartment of the subtalar joint from the lateral and the medial side. Secure the long flexor tendon of the toes while removing the cartilage from the medial side. Check the correction manually. If this is not possible, resect a laterally based wedge from the subtalar joint. Refresh the bone with a drill or a chisel to promote the bony fusion. Close the osteotomy, check the foot shape and axis, and use two 2.5-mm to 3.0-mm K wires for stabilization of every joint. Use the resected cancellous bone to refill the osteotomy defect zones.

Triple fusion with Lambrinudi procedure

Indication:

The indication for triple fusion with Lambrinudi procedure (**Fig. 1**) is severe hindfoot varus with bony ventral dorsiflexion impingement by the talar head and neck on the ventral tibia.[6–10]

- The principle of the Lambrinudi fusion corresponds with the triple fusion.
- In cases of anterior tibiotalar impingement, an anterior-based wedge has to be resected. Two osteotomies of the bone are used. First, the incision with the oscillating saw runs parallel to the ankle joint from anterior and ends in the posterior edge of the subtalar joint. The second osteotomy runs parallel to the subtalar joint line through the calcaneus. While resecting, at least 50% of the talar head should be preserved. The line of the resection of both bony parts should be plane to avoid defect zones after osteotomy closing. Use 2 K wires for osteotomy stabilization.

Lateral closed Dwyer osteotomy

Indication:

The Dwyer osteotomy is used in varus hindfoot, when subtalar arthrodesis is not indicated or the hindfoot cannot be completely reduced. The anatomy of the hindfoot is not affected by the extra-articular osteotomy.[11–13]

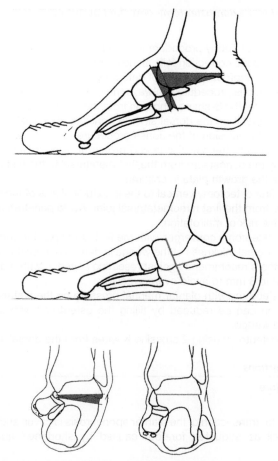

Fig. 1. Triple arthrodesis with additional Lambrinudi procedure. An anterior-based and lateral-based wedge is resected in cases of severe hindfoot varus and anterior tibiotalar impingement.

- The incision is 5 cm perpendicular to the longitudinal axis of the calcaneus directly posterior to the peroneal tendons. After retracting the subcutaneous tissue, protect the sural nerve. Expose the surface of the calcaneus subperiostally.
- Create a laterally based wedge with an oscillating saw. Depending on the varus deformity, the minimal thickness of the wedge should be 5 mm, the maximal thickness 10 mm.
- Penetration of the medial cortex should be avoided to minimize the risk of malrotation and to use the hinge effect. The part of the calcaneus with the insertion of the Achilles tendon should be mobile. The surface of the osteotomy has to be plane to close the osteotomy and to avoid defect zones.
- Resect the wedge, close the osteotomy, and stabilize the osteotomy with 2 K wires. If there is a defect zone, fill it with the cancellous bone from the resected wedge.

First metatarsal dorsiflexion osteotomy described by Tubby

Indication:

The indication for the Tubby procedure is fixed plantarflexion of the first metatarsal when the soft tissue correction fails alone (Tubby and Jones[14]). Every correction of the structural hindfoot and midfoot deformity has to be done before this procedure. Therefore, this procedure is always the last step in correction of deformity.

- The authors prefer the S-shaped incision from the first metatarsal base to the first interphalangeal joint on the dorsal side. In principle, the incision is the proximal lengthening of the incision of the Jones procedure.
- Mobilize and retract the soft tissue and protect it using 2 Hohmann retractors. Incise sharply the periosteum from the first metatarsal to the first tarsometatarsal joint. Expose the growth plate in children.
- Perform the first osteotomy vertical to the longitudinal axis of the first metatarsal, 0.5 cm distal from the first tarsometatarsal joint. Avoid penetration of the plantar cortex with the risk of malrotation.
- The second osteotomy converges with the first at the plantar cortex. A wedge is created. The dorsal thickness of the wedge is determined by the angle of correction. The authors recommend against resecting a wedge with a dorsal thickness larger than 2 to 3 mm to avoid overcorrection.
- Close the osteotomy with plantar manual pressure on the first metatarsal head. Overcorrection can be reduced by filling the osteotomy with spongiosa from the resected wedge.
- Secure the osteotomy using 2 crossing K wires from the dorsal side.

Soft Tissue Corrections

Steindler procedure

Indication:

The indication for transection of the plantar aponeurosis is cavus and equinus deformity, as well as adducted forefoot caused by shortened abductor hallucis tendon.[15,16]

- The incision is on the medial border of the foot, above the insertion point of the plantar aponeurosis at the calcaneus. The insertion is slightly convex and has a length of 3 to 4 cm.
- Divide the subcutaneous tissue from the aponeurosis.
- Insert Langenbeck retractors between the plantar aponeurosis and the fatty tissue of the heel to get the best overview of the plantar aponeurosis.
- Transect the plantar aponeurosis sharply as near to the bone as possible with a scissors. The authors avoid the transection of the long plantar ligament because this runs the risk of an overcorrection.
- In cases of severe cavus deformity, the contemporaneous transection of the short flexor digitorum muscle can be necessary.

Total split posterior tibial tendon transfer

Indication:

The T-SPOTT (**Fig. 2**) is a modified Codivilla procedure.[17] The purpose of this procedure is to substitute dorsiflexors that are weak or absent and to eliminate the pathologic hyperactivity of the posterior tibial muscle with increased inversion. The correction of foot deformity with sufficient range of motion in the ankle joint should be done before or simultaneously. The activity level of the posterior tibial muscle has to be grade 4 or higher before tendon transposition.

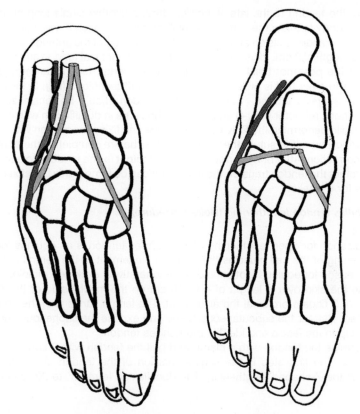

Fig. 2. Principle of the total split posterior tibialis tendon transfer.

- Incise the skin and the subcutaneous tissue to a length of 3 to 4 cm from the medial malleolus to the insertion of the tibialis posterior tendon on the navicular bone. Retract the tissue and expose the flexor retinaculum.
- Incise the sheath of the posterior tibial tendon and cut the tendon nearly to the bony border. In cases of adhesion, use a clamp to undermine the tendon for release.
- The next step is the anterior incision 4 fingerbreadths proximally to the ankle. The bony landmark is the posterior edge of the tibia. Incise and retract the subcutaneous tissue with Langenbeck retractors. Next identify the long toe flexor tendon. The posterior tibial tendon is deep to the long toe flexor tendon. Incise the deep fascia and retract the posterior tibial tendon with a clamp.
- Hold the retracted tendon with a clamp and split it into 2 strands with a scalpel and tag each strand with Vicryl sutures.
- Perform an incision on the lateral side, parallel to the medial incision at the same height in front of the fibula. Incise and retract the subcutaneous fascia while protecting the superficial peroneal nerve. Push a clamp through the interosseous membrane from medial to lateral, and pull a suture loop to the medial incision while protecting the nerves and vessels. Thread the split tendon with the tag sutures in the loop and pull the tendons to the lateral incision. Before the complete

pull of the tendon to the lateral incision, thread another single loop around the tendon body to allow the surgeon to pull the tendons back if needed.

- Perform a medial incision at the height of the insertion of the anterior tibial tendon over a length of 3 cm. Incise the sheath of the anterior tibial tendon and pass one-half of the posterior tibial tendon using the Pulvertaft technique through each other. The other half is pulled using the Pulvertaft technique (**Fig. 3**) through the peroneus brevis tendon. The augmented tendon should be tensioned with a single-hook retractor (**Fig. 4**) and the foot should be in dorsiflexion with extended toes while performing the Pulvertaft technique and fixing the tendon with sutures.
- It is important not to suture these to each other before completing the bony hind-foot correction. After bony correction of the hindfoot fix the tendons to each other. To protect the tendon transfer, the ankle joint can be temporarily transfixed with K wires for 6 weeks.

Open Achilles tendon lengthening (Hoke procedure)

Indication:

The indication for open lengthening of the Achilles tendon is an equinus foot with shortening of the calf muscles.[18] A bony impingement of the ventral ankle joint as a reason for equinus foot should be preoperatively excluded radiologically.

- Incise the skin over a length of 4 to 10 cm on the medial side of the Achilles tendon, 2 fingers proximal the ankle joint. The length varies with the correction needed. Retract the subcutaneous tissue and expose the saphenous nerve and vein. Open the fascia and identify the Achilles tendon.
- Undermine the tendon with a clamp and pull the tendon with 2 Langenbeck retractors. The first step is the sagittal incision of the tendon, and the second step is the Z-shaped lengthening. The dorsiflexion from 10° to 20° should then

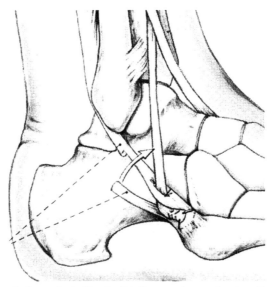

Fig. 3. Pulvertaft technique; the half-split tibialis posterior tendon is pulled through the peroneus brevis tendon (*arrow*). Both tendons are sutured and fixed to each other.

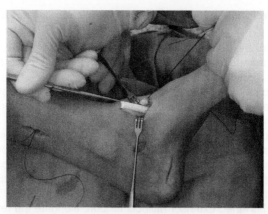

Fig. 4. The anterior tibial tendon is pulled out and tensioned with a single hook retractor. The posterior tibial tendon is sutured to pass one-half of the tendon through the sheath of the anterior tibial tendon. The tibial posterior tendon was pulled out from its origin through the medial tibial incision, which is seen in the left of the picture.

be possible with smooth manual pressure on the plantar side. The ends of the tendon slide apart.

- Tag both ends of the tendon with Vicryl sutures, then suture them together with a side-to-side technique with neutral positioning of the ankle joint.
- Check the tension of the calf muscles. The resistance during manual dorsiflexion should be springy and elastic.

Baumann procedure for hindfoot equinus

Indication:

The correction of structural equinus foot requires the Baumann procedure.[19,20] Mostly this technique concerns patients with previously lengthened Achilles tendon or cerebral palsy. Performing passive bending of the knee, the correction of the foot in the ankle joint is only possible to the neutral position. The purpose of the technique is the incision of the aponeurosis of the gastrocnemius and soleus muscles. The muscle is lengthened without interruption of this structure.

- Perform a 5-cm to 8-cm incision on the medial side of the proximal third of the medial gastrocnemius muscle 1 finger dorsal to the medial edge of the tibia. Retract the subcutaneous tissue and expose the saphenous nerve and vein. Incise the common fascia of the muscles in longitudinal axis.
- Identify the interval between soleus and medial gastrocnemius muscle and open it in longitudinal axis. Check the course of both muscles during passive movement of the ankle joint. Insert 2 Langenbeck retractors to get the best overview.
- Identify and mobilize the cutaneous sural nerve, which often is on the dorsal surface of the medial gastrocnemius muscle between fascia and muscle. Perform a diagonal intramuscular recession of the gastrocnemius aponeurosis. In cases of insufficient correction (intraoperative Silfverskiöld Test), recess the soleus aponeurosis in the same way. The recession should include the complete aponeurosis to the lateral border.
- The ankle joint can then be dorsiflexed and the aponeurosis will slide apart.

Modified Jones procedure with fusion of the hallux interphalangeal joint

Indication:

The indication for the Jones procedure is a clawing hallux.[21,22] The purpose of this procedure is to reduce or eliminate the overactive long extensor hallucis and long flexor hallucis muscles and to achieve an active elevation of the first metatarsal.

- The authors prefer the S-shaped incision from the first metatarsal base to the first interphalangeal joint on the dorsal side. Retract the soft tissue and secure the dorsomedial sensory nerve of the hallux.
- Expose the long extensor hallucis tendon and tag the tendon distally with atraumatic Vicryl sutures. Cut the tendon on the point of the insertion, the distal first phalanx, as near to the bony border as possible. Release and mobilize the tendon to the middle of the first metatarsal. Secure the extensor hallucis brevis tendon, which inserts on the base of the proximal phalanx from lateral.
- In cases of shortened extensor hallucis tendon, elongate the tendon and incise the capsule of the first metatarsophalangeal joint from dorsal and lateral directions to reach plantar flexion.
- To perform arthrodesis of the hallux interphalangeal joint, open the joint capsule and remove the cartilage from the joint. The spongiosa should be completely exposed and drilled to promote joint fusion. Drill 2 K wires crosswise in an antegrade direction through the distal fragment. Then change the position of the power drill on the distal aspect of the K wires. Next drill in a retrograde direction from distal to proximal through both fragments and reduce the joint. Avoid joint extension and malrotation, which carry the risk of postoperative problems with shoe wear. Use 1.4-mm wires in children and 1.8-mm wires in adults. Fill possible defect zones with cancellous bone.
- In the next step, incise the periosteum from the proximal end of the first metatarsal to the middle third of its shaft in a longitudinal direction. If the plantarflexion is not possible by soft tissue correction, extend the procedure and perform a dorsiflexion osteotomy (as discussed for the first metatarsal dorsiflexion osteotomy according to Tubby and Jones[14]).
- Expose the bone, release the periosteum with an elevator, and retract the soft tissue by placing 2 Hohmann retractors. Create a drill hole exactly in the first metatarsal head in a transverse direction. The diameter of the drill hole should be enlarged from 2.0 mm to 3.2 mm.
- Pass the drill hole with a wire or a needle from the first interdigital space to the medial side for transport of the tagged long extensor hallucis tendon.
- Pull the tendon through the drill hole and suture it to itself with an additional Vicryl suture. If the hallux trends to plantar flexion after this procedure, reattach the sutures of the tendon to the periosteum to avoid plantar flexion.

Russel-Hibbs procedure

Indication:

The purpose of the Russel-Hibbs procedure is the soft tissue correction of claw toe deformity.[23] The deformity results from muscular overactivity of the extrinsic muscles (extensor digitorum longus, flexor digitorum longus) and weakness of the intrinsic muscles. The principle of the procedure is the proximal shift of the long extensor digitorum tendons.

- Make a convex dorsal incision in line with the base of the fourth metatarsal to the base of the calcaneocuboid joint with a length of 4 cm. Incise the subcutaneous tissue and expose the superficial peroneal nerve, secure it with a loop, and retract the nerve to the lateral side.

- Expose the long extensor digitorum tendons from the second to the fourth toes. Undermine the tendons with a clamp and tag these together proximally and distally with Vicryl sutures. Then cut the tendons between the 2 sutures.
- Release the extensor digitorum brevis muscle and retract it to the lateral side or incise the muscle in longitudinal axis to expose the lateral cuneiform.
- Incise the periosteum of the lateral cuneiform. In children, the tendons can be sutured to the periosteum. The foot should come into neutral position. Avoid overcorrection to calcaneal foot. In adults, the tendons should be fixed into the bone. The easiest way is the use of a bone anchor.

Complications and management

- A nonunion and malunion of the bony fusion with loss of correction mostly require revision surgery with osteosynthesis of the foot and the use of autologous bone graft from the iliac crest.
- Talus avascular necrosis after extended resection (ie, Lambrinudi procedure).
- An overcorrection of the foot requires either custom-made shoes and braces or revision surgery with plantigrade positioning of the foot.
- Infection with necrosis of the wound can be treated conservatively using special wound management. In rare cases with extended wound necrosis, there is the indication for revision surgery using a vacuum system. Rarely, plastic surgery is required.
- Compression of the nerves and vessels can occur because of increased tension of surrounding soft tissue.
- Failure of the tendon transfer. In these cases, the treatment can be conservative with a brace. In cases of loss of correction of the foot after rupture of the tendon, revision surgery is indicated to perform another tendon transfer (ie, Hiroshima procedure with transfer of the long flexor digitorum tendon).

Postoperative care

- The authors prefer to use a drain for each wound, leaving it in for 2 days. During this time, the foot is fixed in a cardboard splint in neutral position for 2 days.
- From this time on, weight bearing is completely restricted for 6 weeks.
- On the second day, the cardboard splint is removed, the dressings are changed, and a short-leg fiberglass cast is applied for 2 weeks.
- After 2 weeks, the patient gets a short-leg fiberglass cast and all sutures are removed.
- At the follow-up after 6 weeks, new radiographs are obtained. According to the status of the bony fusion, the K wires are removed. The patient gets a new short-leg fiberglass cast with a sole. Weight bearing is restricted to 20 kg until the ninth week.
- At the follow-up after 9 weeks, there is a new radiographic control. The patient gets a new short-leg fiberglass cast, which can be removed while resting.
- At the 12-week follow-up, the patient gets a final radiograph. According to the bony fusion, the cast can be removed completely. Depending on the severity of the deformity and the neurologic conditions, the authors recommend to wear a splint for another 6 months.

Outcomes with illustrative cases

- Three cases are presented as examples of the principles described earlier.

- The first case shows a 34-year-old man with Charcot-Marie-Tooth disease and equinocavovarus deformity on both sides. The clinical and radiological examination showed hindfoot varus and equinus, cavus deformity, and plantarflexion of the first metatarsal with concomitant claw toes on both sides (**Fig. 5**A, B). The surgical treatment was a triple arthrodesis, Jones procedure, a T-SPOTT, dorsiflexion osteotomy of the first metatarsal, Steindler procedure, and lengthening of the Achilles tendon. Six weeks after the primary surgery, the contralateral side was done in the same way. The postoperative results are shown in **Fig. 5**C–E. Six months postoperatively, the patient went back to his job.
- The second case shows a 47-year-old man with congenital clubfoot on the right side. The clinical examination showed an equinovarus et adductus with tight

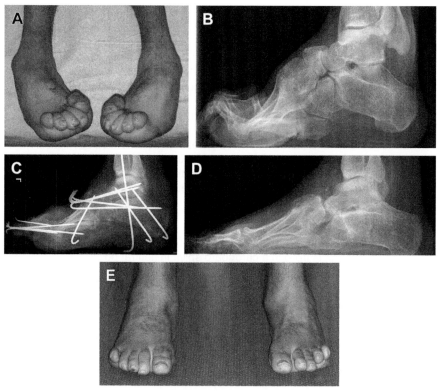

Fig. 5. Preoperative clinical (*A*) and radiographic (*B*) findings of the left side of a 28-year-old man with Charcot-Marie-Tooth disease. The patient shows an equinocavovarus deformity on both sides with severe clawing toes, including a clawing hallux, external rotated fibula, and prominent base of the 5th metatarsus in the lateral radiographic view. In the same patient, postoperative radiographic findings (*C, D*) and clinical findings (*E*). The procedure was triple arthrodesis with extraction of the navicular bone to reach correction and a nearly plantigrade foot axis on both sides. In addition, the total split posterior tibial tendon transfer was performed to support the active dorsiflexion and to eliminate the pathologic inversion of each foot. To reduce the clawing hallux, the modified Jones procedure was done with dorsiflexion osteotomy. In addition, the Steindler procedure was performed. Furthermore, the external rotation of the ankle joint could be corrected by this procedure.

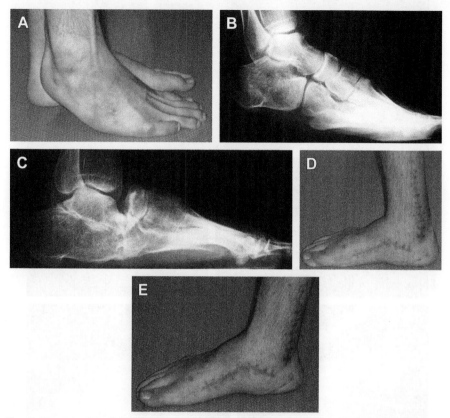

Fig. 6. Preoperative clinical (*A*) and radiographic (*B*) findings of a 23-year-old man with congenital clubfoot and equinovarus et adductus deformity on the right side. The lateral radiographic view shows an external rotated ankle joint and a prominent fifth metatarsus. In the same patient, postoperative radiographic findings (*C*) and clinical findings (*D, E*) in dorsiflexion and plantarflexion after triple arthrodesis with Lambrinudi procedure, total split posterior tibialis tendon transfer, and lengthening of the Achilles tendon.

extensor digitorum longus tendon. The surgical treatment was a triple arthrodesis and Lambrinudi procedure for correction of hindfoot varus and bony limitation of dorsiflexion. Furthermore, the T-SPOTT and lengthening of the Achilles tendon were performed surgically. A nearly plantigrade foot was restored (**Fig. 6**).

- The third case shows a 30-year-old man with postpolio foot. The clinical examination showed a complete malrotation of the subtalar joint with severe equinovarus deformity. The surgical procedure was a triple arthrodesis with Lambrinudi procedure. The reason for the Lambrinudi procedure was the severe hindfoot varus and massive deformity of the hindfoot and midfoot. In addition to the bony correction, a tendon transfer was performed to balance the foot. A nearly plantigrade foot was restored. After 6 months and intensive physical treatment, the patient went back to his job (**Fig. 7**).

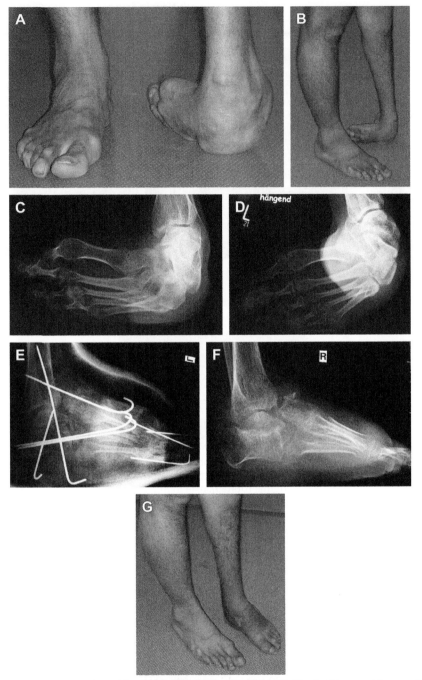

Fig. 7. Preoperative clinical (*A, B*) and radiological findings (*C, D*) of a 30-year-old man with postpolio clubfoot on the left side. The complete midfoot and hindfoot are malrotated to each other. The center of rotation angle of the deformity is the Chopart and the subtalar joint. (*C*) AP view. (*D*) Lateral view on the ankle joint. The position of the midfoot relative to the forefoot is acceptable. The surgical procedure was a triple arthrodesis with Lambrinudi procedure. The reason for a Lambrinudi procedure was the severe hindfoot varus and massive deformity of the hindfoot and midfoot. The first radiograph (*E*) was taken after 6 weeks, and the second (*F*) after 12 weeks. In summary, the patient received a nearly plantigrade, shoeable foot (*G*). There is no loss of correction.

SUMMARY

The severely deformed foot with neurologic conditions that cannot fit into normal shoes or that results in an impossible physiologic gait presents a challenge for foot surgeons. This article shows that a variety of deformities can be approached with the same principles. The focus is always on the bony fusion of the midfoot and additionally the hindfoot in severe cases, which is the center of rotation angle of the deformity in most cases. The authors prefer the use of removable K wires for 6 weeks after surgery. The purpose of this procedure is the use of the physiologic bone biology for the healing process and to prevent bony compression with screws.

In our view, simple tendon transfers and soft tissue correction in severe foot deformities are not sufficient and are accompanied by recurrence rates. The authors use soft tissue correction principles only in addition to bony fusions to balance the foot.

REFERENCES

1. Coleman SS, Chesnut WJ. A simple test for hindfoot flexibility in the cavovarus foot. Clin Orthop Relat Res 1977;(123):60–2.
2. Akinci O, Akalin Y. Medium-term results of single-stage posteromedial release and triple arthrodesis in treatment of neglected clubfoot deformity in adults. Acta Orthop Traumatol Turc 2015;49:175–83.
3. Hoke M. An operation for stabilizing paralytic feet. J Orthop Surg 1921;3:494.
4. Imhauser G. Early treatment of congenital, muscular clubfoot. Monatsschr Kinderheilkd 1969;117:645–8 [in German].
5. Imhauser G. Surgical treatment of severe talipes cavus and ball arcuatus. Z Orthop Ihre Grenzgeb 1969;106:488–94 [in German].
6. Benyi PA. modified Lambrinudi operation for drop foot. J Bone Joint Surg Br 1960; 42-B:333–5.
7. Elsner A, Barg A, Stufkens S, et al. Modified Lambrinudi arthrodesis with additional posterior tibial tendon transfer in adult drop foot. Oper Orthop Traumatol 2011;23:121–30 [in German].
8. Hall JE, Calvert PT. Lambrinudi triple arthrodesis: a review with particular reference to the technique of operation. J Pediatr Orthop 1987;7:19–24.
9. Lambrinudi C. New operation on drop-foot. Br J Surg 1927;15:193–200.
10. Schwetlick G, Syre F. Severe foot deformities in adolescents and adults–techniques after Imhauser, Lelievre und Lambrinudi. Orthopade 2006;35:422–7 [in German].
11. Csizy M, Hintermann B. Dwyer osteotomy with or without lateral stabilization in calcaneus varus with lateral ligament insufficiency of the upper ankle joint. Sportverletz Sportschaden 1996;10:100–2 [in German].
12. Dwyer FC. Osteotomy of the calcaneum for pes cavus. J Bone Joint Surg Br 1959;41-B:80–6.
13. Robinson DS, Clark B Jr, Prigoff MM. Dwyer osteotomy for treatment of calcaneal varus. J Foot Surg 1988;27:541–4.
14. Tubby AH, Jones R. Modern methods in the surgery of the paralysis. London: MacMillan; 1903.
15. Fulford GE. Surgical management of ankle and foot deformities in cerebral palsy. Clin Orthop Relat Res 1990;(253):55–61.
16. Steindler A. The treatment of pes cavus (hollow claw foot). Arch Surg 1921;2: 325–37.

17. Hsu JD, Hoffer MM. Posterior tibial tendon transfer anteriorly through the interosseous membrane: a modification of the technique. Clin Orthop Relat Res 1978;(131):202–4.

18. Hoke M. An operation for the correction of extremely relaxed feet. J Bone Joint Surg 1931;13:773–83.

19. Baumann JU. Treatment of pediatric spastic foot deformities. Orthopade 1986;15: 191–8 [in German].

20. Baumann J. Operative Behandlung der infantilen Cerebralparese. Stuttgart (Germany); New York: Thieme; 1970.

21. Giannini S, Girolami M, Ceccarelli F, et al. Modified Jones operation in the treatment of pes cavovarus. Ital J Orthop Traumatol 1985;11:165–70.

22. Jones R. An operation for paralytic calcanoe-cavus. Am J Orthop Surg 1908;5: 371–6.

23. Hibbs R. An operation for "claw foot". JAMA 1919;73:1583–5.

Recent Advances in Foot and Ankle Surgery in Mainland China

Correction of Severe Foot and Ankle Deformities

Yuan Zhu, MD, Xiang-yang Xu, MD*, Bi-bo Wang, MD

KEYWORDS

- Foot ankle deformity • Severe • Staged surgery • Varus ankle • Ankle arthritis

KEY POINTS

- Foot and ankle physicians in China encounter quite a large amount of severe deformities.
- The preoperative assessment is critical, including where the deformity lies, whether there exists multiplanar deformities, and how much muscle strength there is.
- A staged procedure is a safer way to correct deformities in the presence of severe soft tissue contracture.
- Periarticular osteotomy combined with soft tissue balancing can be used in treating severe varus ankle arthritis, including stage IIIb cases and patients with talar tilt of more than 10°.

THE SITUATION OF SEVERE FOOT AND ANKLE DEFORMITIES IN PRESENT CHINA

Foot and ankle surgery is a young yet dynamically developing specialty in China. The Chinese Foot and Ankle Society was established in 1992, and several foot and ankle centers emerged afterward. With the accumulation of professional knowledge and surgical skills, the scope and volume of foot and ankle surgery have been growing rapidly in the past decades. The advances and experiences in foot and ankle surgery in mainland China are presented in the form of severe ankle and foot deformity correction.

Because there is a large population in China, foot and ankle problems widely exist in various forms and stages. Unfortunately, they were largely neglected in the past when most people were striving for basic life necessities. It is not uncommon to see patients suffering from ankle and foot pain and deformity for as many as 20 to 60 years, mainly because of a poor economic situation and/or lack of proper medical treatment.

The authors have nothing to disclose.
Shanghai Ruijin Hospital, Shanghai Jiaotong university school of medicine, 197 Ruijin Er Road, Shanghai 200025, China
* Corresponding author.
E-mail address: xu664531@hotmail.com

Because the economy in China has grown considerably in the past 30 years, more and more of those patients have the ability to pursue ways to improve their quality of life. They are willing to undergo surgery to correct their long-time deformity to relieve the pain and improve their function as well as appearance.

There are several causes of severe foot and ankle deformity. Trauma is the main cause of severe ankle and foot deformity.[1,2] Some trauma is the result of improper reduction and fixation; others are results of not having any treatment at all. Besides trauma, neuromuscular diseases, such as poliomyelitis, tethered cord syndrome, Charcot-Marie-Tooth (CMT) disease, spinal cord injury, stroke, also cause severe ankle and foot deformity and loss of function. New cases of polio have disappeared in China recently, but there are still many adult patients suffering with residual lower limb deformities due to polio from decades before.

CLINICAL EVALUATION OF SEVERE FOOT AND ANKLE DEFORMITIES

A weight-bearing physical examination is an important method for evaluating the deformities of the foot and ankle.[3,4] In this position, the physician can observe the hindfoot varus/valgus, the twist of the midfoot, and the real height of the foot arch. The deformity may not be isolated to the foot and ankle, so the physical examination should include the whole affected lower limb and compare the affected with the unaffected side. If there has been prior trauma or surgery proximal to the ankle level, the whole alignment of the affected extremity should be inspected and measured carefully. Every single muscle tendon across the ankle should be evaluated carefully, and the muscle power should be recorded so that the muscle balancing plan can be made preoperatively in detail. Active and passive range of motion of the ankle, subtalar joint, as well as the joints of the midfoot should be examined. The authors use the anterior drawer test to evaluate the stability of the ankle.

Weight-bearing radiography is a fundamental radiologic examination.[3–9] In the case of deformities proximal to the ankle level, weight-bearing full-length radiographs from hip to ankle should be obtained. As to the evaluation of hindfoot alignment, the authors recommend the Saltzman hindfoot axis view.[10,11] Computed tomographic (CT) scan with image reconstruction is useful to determine the rotational deformity of the talus, the details of the bony structures, or whether the old fracture has healed. MRI can be used to show the range of the involved articular cartilage.

THE SURGICAL TREATMENT OF SEVERE FOOT AND ANKLE DEFORMITIES

Treatment strategy is summarized as follows. (1) An attempt is made to preserve the ankle if possible. Indications of preserving the ankle lie in that the articular cartilage remains greater than 50% according to MRI; the range of motion of the ankle reaches at least 10° dorsiflexion and 30° plantar flexion. The deformities can be corrected by realignment procedures. (2) Osteotomy or fusion of the Chopart joints may correct the cavovarus deformity, hindfoot malalignment, and midfoot adduction from multiplanes. (3) If the articular cartilage is severely impaired or unbalanced, muscle strength is ill-fated, and the joint-sparing procedure must be abandoned.[12,13] **Fig. 1** (case 1) shows the correction of a severe pes equino-cavovarus case. (4) For those with very severe varus or valgus deformity, an external fixator can be used to correct the deformity in a tender and gradual way in order to protect the neurovascular bundle before the definite procedure. Staged surgery is a safer way of handling severe or complex deformities. Cases in point are shown in **Figs. 2** and **3** (case 2 and case 3).

The sequence of the procedures of correcting the severe equinocavovarus deformity of the foot and ankle is usually performed by: (a) release of the medial and

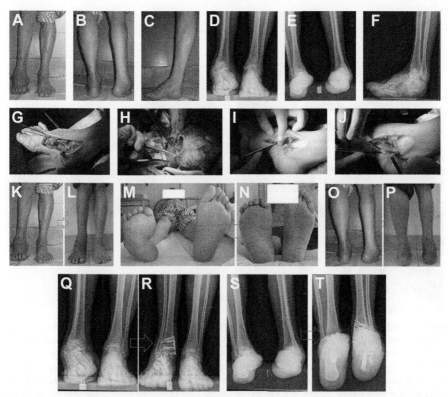

Fig. 1. Case 1: A 58-year-old man who suffered from poliomyelitis 50 years ago. (*A–F*) Pre-operative appearance and radiograph show pes equino-cavo-varus deformity. (*G, H*) Bony correction: supramalleolar osteotomy + calcaneal lateralizing osteotomy + talo-navicular joint reduction and fusion + calcaneo-cuboidal joint fusion + 1st and 2nd metatarsal dorsal flexion osteotomy. (*I, J*) Soft tissue balance: ankle joint clearance + Achilles tendon lengthening + medial contractive tissue release + anterior tibial tendon transfer to middle cuneiform + PTT transferred to the base of the 5th metatarsal. (*K–T*) Preoperative versus 4 months postoperative: pes equino-cavo-varus deformity corrected.

posterior soft tissues such as the Achilles tendon, the flexors (posterior tibial tendon [PTT], flexor hallucis longus [FHL], flexor digitorum longus [FDL]), and/or the posterior capsule of the ankle. Sometimes the Z lengthening of the spring ligament is performed in patients with severe medial soft tissue contracture. Osteophytes are removed at the same time. The goal of these procedures is to put the ankle back to its proper position so that a congruent ankle joint is achieved. (b) The joints are realigned by supramalleolar osteotomy, calcaneal osteotomy, and/or Chopart joint osteotomy. (c) Augmentations or reconstruction of the ligaments is performed (such as modified Broström, Chrisman-Snook procedure, autograft/allograft anatomic reconstruction). (d) Tendon transfer may be performed to balance the muscle power.

THE SURGICAL TREATMENT OF SEVERE VARUS ANKLE ARTHRITIS

Improper primary treatment of ankle fracture can result in late deformity and malfunction. Neglected ligament injury may develop into chronic ankle instability, which is also a cause of ankle osteoarthritis (OA) with talar tilt.[4,14–18]

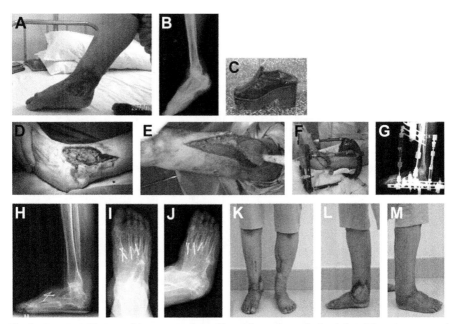

Fig. 2. Case 2: A 60-year-old woman who suffered from an explosive injury 40 years ago, and chronic infection since then. (*A*) She presented with an equinus deformity of the right foot and large area of unhealed infectious ulcer at the medial ankle. (*B*) Lateral radiograph film of the ankle. (*C*) High-heel shoe constructed to accommodate the equinus deformity. (*D*) The ulcer and scar at the medial ankle were resected, and the medial soft tissue was released. (*E*) To cover the soft tissue defect, a sural nerve island flap pedicled with collateral vessels was transplanted. (*F, G*) An external fixator was applied to correct the equinus deformity gradually and to protect the surgical flap. (*H–J*) The 2nd stage surgery: osteotomy of the 1st to 3rd metatarsal to correct the forefoot and midfoot supination. (*K–M*) The general appearance of the foot and ankle 5 months after the 2nd operation showed that the long-time severely deformed foot and ankle were fully corrected to a plantigrade foot.

There are various single or combined surgical procedures in the treatment of varus ankle OA. Tibiotalar fusion remains the mainstay for most surgeons around the world in treating end-stage ankle arthritis,[19,20] although complications like infection, nonunion, or adjacent-joint arthritis may hamper the final outcome.[21–23] Because many patients of ankle OA feel pain intermittently, they do not want to lose the ankle joint. Total ankle replacement can preserve the motion of the ankle and relieve the pain in patients with ankle arthritis,[24,25] and it is performed in several foot and ankle centers in China. However, because of commerce concerns, the prosthesis has not been available in China until recently. Thus, osteotomy around the ankle has been performed for pain relief and deformity correction. There are some preconditions for the patients selected for the osteotomy correction of ankle OA, such as proper range of motion of the ankle and 50% or more articular cartilage remaining.[26–29]

It has been described by several physicians that the supramalleolar osteotomy cannot be applied for stage IIIb ankles according to the Takakura classification or tilting talus greater than 10°.[4,29–31] Because many patients have a strong desire to preserve their ankle joint motion and the prosthesis for ankle arthroplasty has not been

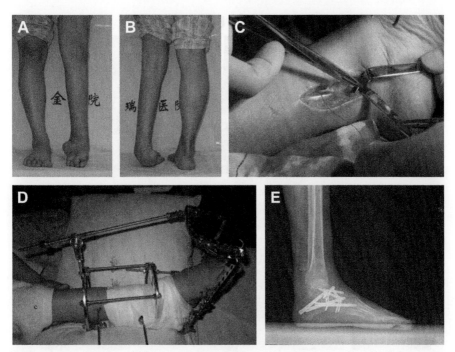

Fig. 3. Case 3: a 31-year-old female patient with a severe varus foot and ankle due to polio. (*A*) and (*B*) The appearance before surgical treatment. (*C*) Stage 1 surgery included soft tissue release and external fixation. The frame was used to correct the deformity gradually and safely. The aim of limited open soft tissue surgery (achilles tendon [AT], PTT, FHL, FDL lengthening) was to save time of external fixation. (*D*) The frame was removed 2 months later, after the varus deformity had been corrected. (*E*) Because of the degenerated change of the joints, a triple arthrodesis was ultimately performed.

available in the Chinese market for very long, the authors try to treat deformity with osteotomies and debridement around the ankle, along with other procedures if necessary, for patients of stage II–III ankle OA. The joint-preserving procedures were performed on those with or without talar tilting to correct deformity and relieve pain (**Fig. 4**, case 4).

Sometimes there are additional deformities above the ankle. The proximal deformities should be corrected before the ankle surgery or be handled simultaneously in order to realign the mechanical axis (**Fig. 5**, case 5).

The authors have participated in a midterm retrospective study of periarticular osteotomy in treating severe asymmetric ankle arthritis. The periarticular osteotomy includes supramalleolar osteotomy and calcaneal osteotomy. Forty-two sequential cases were collected between 2009 and 2012. The age of surgery ranged from 31 to 70 years (mean, 55.5). According to the Takakura classification of ankle arthritis, there were 16 cases in grade IIIa and 26 cases in grade IIIb. The average follow-up time was 44.5 months (36–75 months). All patients got complete bone healing with an average healing time of 8 weeks. Average postoperative American Orthopaedic Foot and Ankle Society (AOFAS)-Hind-foot and Ankle (HA) score by the last follow-up was 76.6 (compared with 35.7 preoperatively). Delayed wound healing occurred in 5 cases and was solved with wound care. Of the 26 cases in

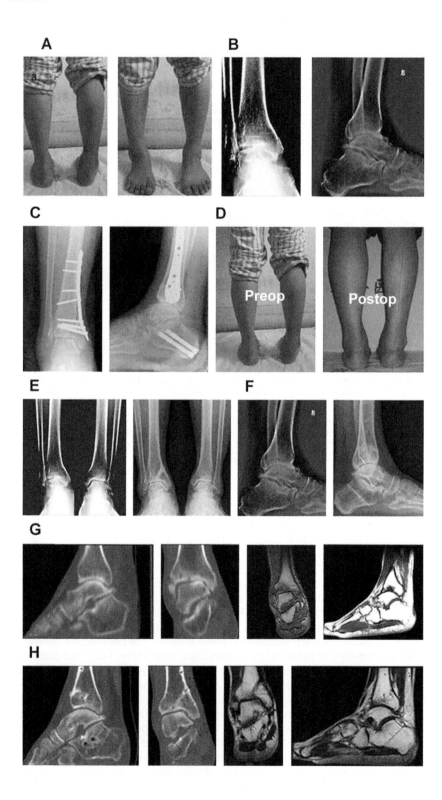

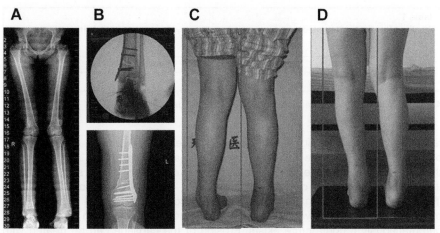

Fig. 5. Case 5: a 40-year-old female patient demonstrated a valgus knee and a varus ankle at the left lower extremity. (*A*) The whole lower extremities weight-bearing radiograph examination showed a valgus knee and varus ankle deformity on the left side. (*B*) An open wedge osteotomy above the left knee was performed to correct the valgus knee deformity, and a medial supramalleolar osteotomy was performed to correct the varus ankle deformity. A triple arthrodesis was done simultaneously to treat the degenerative change of the hindfoot. (*C, D*) The patient's alignment of her left lower limb was corrected after the osteotomies.

grade IIIb, the Takakura ankle arthritis grade went down to grade I in 5 cases, grade II in 19 cases, and grade IIIa in 2 cases. All 16 cases in grade IIIa downgraded to I. All the cases had improvements in Takakura ankle arthritis classification by the last follow-up after surgery. Twenty-two of the 42 patients thought the result was excellent, and 20 of the 42 thought the result was good. The most significant improvement experience from the patients was the pain release. The radiological assessment by the last follow-up also showed improvement by more congruent joint, wider joint space, and less degenerative changes. By the last follow-up, none of these patients received or wanted to receive further surgeries, such as ankle arthrodesis or ankle replacement (see **Fig. 4**; **Table 1**).

The procedures below the level of the ankle, such as calcaneal osteotomy and lateral ligament reconstruction, may not correct the tibiotalar varus deformity successfully. The ankle tends to fall back into varus afterward; this may be caused by erosion of the medial plafond as a result of the chronic varus malposition of the

Fig. 4. Case 4: a 63-year-old male patient with asymmetric ankle arthritis. (*A*) This patient presented a varus ankle deformity. (*B*) Radiograph examination showed a varus and incongruent ankle (with a talar tilt of 19°) from the anteroposterior view and narrow space of the ankle from the lateral view. (*C*) An oblique supramalleolar osteotomy, a calcaneal osteotomy, and a lateral ligament augmentation (modified Broström) were performed. (*D–F*) The results of 5-year postoperative follow-up compared with his preoperative conditions (*left*: preoperative appearance and radiograph demonstration; *right*: 5 years postoperative results). The Takakura classification was downgraded from IIIb to I. (*G*) The preoperative CT scan and MRI findings. (*H*) The CT scan and MRI findings 4 years after surgery. The CT scan showed the ankle joint became more congruent and the space of the joint wider. The degenerative change of the ankle improved from the MRI findings.

Table 1
Results of periarticular osteotomy in treating severe asymmetric ankle arthritis

	TAS	VAS Score	AOFAS Score
Before surgery	86.1°±°2.2	7.9°±°1.5	35.7°±°5.6
Last follow-up after surgery	93.9°±°1.0	1.6°±°1.3	76.6°±°4.4

Abbreviations: TAS, tibial anterior surface angle; VAS, visual analog scale.

talus.[15,32–35] The investigators start with ankle clearance and supramalleolar osteotomy to reduce the talus and shift the load to the lateral side.[36–38] After that, the alignment of the ankle and hindfoot is evaluated by the surgeon during the surgery in order to decide if an additional calcaneal osteotomy is needed (**Fig. 6**). The lateral ligament augmentation or reconstruction procedure is often needed in cases with talar tilt.[32,39–41] The Achilles tendon is lengthened percutaneously if contracture exists. Erosion of the cartilage can be treated with a microfracture.

According to midterm follow-up, periarticular osteotomy is a sound method in treating asymmetric ankle arthritis. Even the Takakura classification of IIIb patients can benefit from this method. The alignment of the joint and the axis of whole lower limb are the most important factors related to the final result. The severity of talar tilt before surgery seems not to be a factor as was previously thought. However, it can lead to poor results if it appears in the weight-bearing radiograph after surgery.

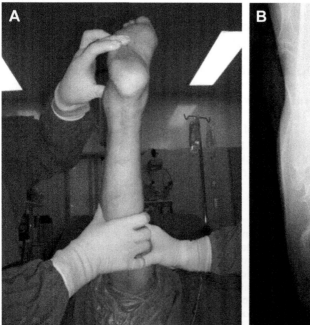
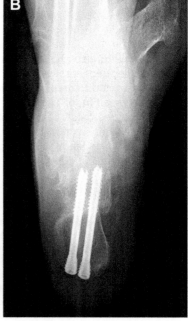

Fig. 6. The alignment of the ankle and hindfoot is evaluated during surgery. (*A*) The surgeon elevated the lower limb by holding the lateral side of the forefoot to evaluate the alignment. (*B*) A calcaneal osteotomy was performed.

SUMMARY

The surgical treatment of severe foot and ankle deformities is challenging. Preoperative assessment is critical, including where the deformity lies, whether there are multiplanar deformities, and how strong the muscle is. Satisfactory outcomes are rarely achieved without comprehensive procedures. The goal of the surgical approach is to correct the malalignment, while gaining a stable and plantigrade foot and ankle with reasonable function.[18,42–45]

A staged procedure with an external frame to correct the deformity gradually followed by a definite open internal fixation is a safer way to treat deformities with severe soft tissue contracture.

Additional deformities proximal to the ankle level should be treated before or during the ankle correction. The goal is to maintain normal alignment of hip-knee-ankle-calcaneus axis.

Periarticular osteotomy combined with soft tissue balancing can be used in selected patients with severe varus ankle arthritis.[42–47] This series of procedures can correct the malalignment and shift the load to a more physiologic situation, which may relieve the symptoms in most patients.

REFERENCES

1. Valderrabano V, Horisberger M, Russell I. Etiology of ankle osteoarthritis. Clin Orthop Relat Res 2009;467(7):1800–6.
2. Weston JT, Liu X, Wandtke ME. A systematic review of total dislocation of the talus. Orthop Surg 2015;7(2):97–101.
3. Queen RM, Carter JE, Adams SB, et al. Coronal plane ankle alignment, gait, and end-stage ankle osteoarthritis. Osteoarthritis Cartilage 2011;19(11):1338–42.
4. Lee WC, Moon JS, Lee HS, et al. Alignment of ankle and hindfoot in early stage ankle osteoarthritis. Foot Ankle Int 2011;32(7):693–9.
5. Barg A, Amendola RL, Henninger HB. Influence of ankle position and radiographic projection angle on measurement of supramalleolar alignment on the anteroposterior and hindfoot alignment views. Foot Ankle Int 2015;36(11): 1352–61.
6. Stufkens SA, Barg A, Bolliger L. Measurement of the medial distal tibial angle. Foot Ankle Int 2011;32(3):288–93.
7. Barg A, Harris MD, Henninger HB. Medial distal tibial angle: comparison between weightbearing mortise view and hindfoot alignment view. Foot Ankle Int 2012; 33(8):655–61.
8. Nosewicz TL, Knupp M, Bolliger L. Radiological morphology of peritalar instability in varus and valgus tilted ankles. Foot Ankle Int 2014;35(5):453–62.
9. Nosewicz TL, Knupp M, Bolliger L, et al. The reliability and validity of radiographic measurements for determining the three-dimensional position of the talus in varus and valgus osteoarthritic ankles. Skeletal Radiol 2012;41(12):1567–73.
10. Frigg A, Nigg B, Davis E, et al. Does alignment in the hindfoot radiograph influence dynamic foot-floor pressures in ankle and tibiotalocalcaneal fusion? Clin Orthop Relat Res 2010;468(12):3362–70.
11. Saltzman CL, el-Khoury GY. The hindfoot alignment view. Foot Ankle Int 1995; 16(9):572–6.
12. Moon JS, Shim JC, Suh JS, et al. Radiographic predictability of cartilage damage in medial ankle osteoarthritis. Clin Orthop Relat Res 2010;468(8):2188–97.
13. Fang Z, Claaßen L, Windhagen H. Tibiotalocalcaneal arthrodesis using a retrograde intramedullary nail with a valgus curve. Orthop Surg 2015;7(2):125–31.

14. Valderrabano V, Hintermann B, Horisberger M, et al. Ligamentous posttraumatic ankle osteoarthritis. Am J Sports Med 2006;34(4):612–20.
15. Hintermann B, Knupp M, Barg A. Joint-preserving surgery of asymmetric ankle osteoarthritis with peritalar instability. Foot Ankle Clin 2013;18(3):503–16.
16. Hintermann B, Knupp M, Barg A. Peritalar instability. Foot Ankle Int 2012;33(5): 450–4.
17. Colin F, Bolliger L, Horn Lang T. Effect of supramalleolar osteotomy and total ankle replacement on talar position in the varus osteoarthritic ankle: a comparative study. Foot Ankle Int 2014;35(5):445–52.
18. Tanaka Y. The concept of ankle joint preserving surgery: why does supramalleolar osteotomy work and how to decide when to do an osteotomy or joint replacement. Foot Ankle Clin 2012;17(4):545–53.
19. Takakura Y, Tanaka Y, Sugimoto K, et al. Long-term results of arthrodesis for osteoarthritis of the ankle. Clin Orthop Relat Res 1999;361:178–85.
20. Colin F, Zwicky L, Barg A. Peritalar instability after tibiotalar fusion for valgus unstable ankle in stage IV adult acquired flatfoot deformity: case series. Foot Ankle Int 2013;34(12):1677–82.
21. Ling JS, Smyth NA, Fraser EJ, et al. Investigating the relationship between ankle arthrodesis and adjacent-joint arthritis in the hindfoot. A systematic review. J Bone Joint Surg Am 2015;97(9):e43.
22. Saltzman CL, Kadoko RG, Suh JS. Treatment of isolated ankle osteoarthritis with arthrodesis or the total ankle replacement: a comparison of early outcomes. Clin Orthop Surg 2010;2(1):1–7.
23. Baumhauer JF. Ankle arthrodesis versus ankle replacement for ankle arthritis. Clin Orthop Relat Res 2013;471(8):2439–42.
24. Daniels TR, Mayich DJ, Penner MJ. Intermediate to long-term outcomes of total ankle replacement with the Scandinavian Total Ankle Replacement (STAR). J Bone Joint Surg Am 2015;97(11):895–903.
25. Gougoulias N, Khanna A, Maffulli N. How successful are current ankle replacements?: a systematic review of the literature. Clin Orthop Relat Res 2010; 468(1):199–208.
26. Knupp M, Stufkens SA, Bolliger L, et al. Classification and treatment of supramalleolar deformities. Foot Ankle Int 2011;32(11):1023–31.
27. Tanaka Y, Takakura Y, Hayashi K, et al. Low tibial osteotomy for varus-type osteoarthritis of the ankle. J Bone Joint Surg Br 2006;88(7):909–13.
28. Takakura Y, Tanaka Y, Kumai T, et al. Low tibial osteotomy for osteoarthritis of the ankle. Results of a new operation in 18 patients. J Bone Joint Surg Br 1995;77(1):50–4.
29. Lee WC, Moon JS, Lee K, et al. Indications for supramalleolar osteotomy in patients with ankle osteoarthritis and varus deformity. J Bone Joint Surg Am 2011; 93(13):1243–8.
30. Lee WC, Ahn JY, Cho JH, et al. Realignment surgery for severe talar tilt secondary to paralytic cavovarus. Foot Ankle Int 2013;34(11):1552–9.
31. Pagenstert GI, Hintermann B, Barg A, et al. Realignment surgery as alternative treatment of varus and valgus ankle osteoarthritis. Clin Orthop Relat Res 2007; 462:156–68.
32. Lee HS, Wapner KL, Park SS, et al. Ligament reconstruction and calcaneal osteotomy for osteoarthritis of the ankle. Foot Ankle Int 2009;30(6):475–80.
33. Myerson MS, Zide JR. Management of varus ankle osteoarthritis with joint-preserving osteotomy. Foot Ankle Clin 2013;18(3):471–80.

34. Stamatis ED, Myerson MS. Supramalleolar osteotomy: indications and technique. Foot Ankle Clin 2003;8(2):317–33.
35. Becker AS, Myerson MS. The indications and technique of supramalleolar osteotomy. Foot Ankle Clin 2009;14(3):549–61.
36. Haraguchi N, Ota K, Tsunoda N. Weight-bearing-line analysis in supramalleolar osteotomy for varus-type osteoarthritis of the ankle. J Bone Joint Surg Am 2015;97(4):333–9.
37. Knupp M, Stufkens SA, van Bergen CJ. Effect of supramalleolar varus and valgus deformities on the tibiotalar joint: a cadaveric study. Foot Ankle Int 2011;32(6): 609–15.
38. Nüesch C, Valderrabano V, Huber C. Effects of supramalleolar osteotomies for ankle osteoarthritis on foot kinematics and lower leg muscle activation during walking. Clin Biomech (Bristol, Avon) 2014;29(3):257–64.
39. Barg A, Pagenstert GI, Horisberger M. Supramalleolar osteotomies for degenerative joint disease of the ankle joint: indication, technique and results. Int Orthop 2013;37(9):1683–95.
40. Knupp M, Hintermann B. Treatment of asymmetric arthritis of the ankle joint with supramalleolar osteotomies. Foot Ankle Int 2012;33(3):250–2.
41. Colin F, Gaudot F, Odri G, et al. Supramalleolar osteotomy: techniques, indications and outcomes in a series of 83 cases. Orthop Traumatol Surg Res 2014; 100(4):413–8.
42. Schmid T, Zurbriggen S, Zderic I, et al. Ankle joint pressure changes in a pes cavovarus model: supramalleolar valgus osteotomy versus lateralizing calcaneal osteotomy. Foot Ankle Int 2013;34(9):1190–7.
43. Krause FG, Henning J, Pfander G, et al. Cavovarus foot realignment to treat anteromedial ankle arthrosis. Foot Ankle Int 2013;34(1):54–64.
44. Ryssman DB, Myerson MS. Tendon transfers for the adult flexible cavovarus foot. Foot Ankle Clin 2011;16(3):435–50.
45. Hogan MV, Dare DM, Deland JT. Is deltoid and lateral ligament reconstruction necessary in varus and valgus ankle osteoarthritis, and how should these procedures be performed? Foot Ankle Clin 2013;18(3):517–27.
46. Irwin TA, Anderson RB, Davis WH, et al. Effect of ankle arthritis on clinical outcome of lateral ankle ligament reconstruction in cavovarus feet. Foot Ankle Int 2010;31(11):941–8.
47. Mann HA, Filippi J, Myerson MS. Intra-articular opening medial tibial wedge osteotomy(plafond-plasty) for the treatment of intra-articular varus ankle arthritis and instability. Foot Ankle Int 2012;33(4):255–61.

Total Toe Replacement in the United States

What Is Known and What Is on the Horizon

Michael D. Johnson, MD[a],*, Michael E. Brage, MD[b]

KEYWORDS

- Total toe arthroplasty • Bipolar toe arthroplasty • Hallux rigidus

KEY POINTS

- There is a high rate of radiologic loosening with arthroplasty implants of the first metatarsophalangeal joint.
- The presence of loosening does not always correlate with patient satisfaction.
- Failed arthroplasties may be treated with fusion with structural bone graft.
- Well-designed and controlled investigations with modern implants are needed to guide treatment recommendations.

INTRODUCTION: NATURE OF THE PROBLEM

Arthritis of first metatarsophalangeal joint can be a painful and debilitating problem and is one of the most common pathologies affecting the forefoot. Patients often present with pain and limited range of motion (ROM) of the first metatarsophalangeal joint. The pain is typically worse with dorsiflexion of the hallux and is exacerbated by prolonged activity. Furthermore, the dorsal osteophyte may cause pain with shoe wear (**Fig. 1**). Patients may also develop lateral forefoot symptoms as patients attempt to off-load the first metatarsophalangeal joint by transferring weight laterally. Patients are often most comfortable in flat shoes because their symptoms are exacerbated with shoes having any elevation of the heel.

Physical examination often reveals pain with ROM along with swelling and tenderness to palpation of the first metatarsophalangeal joint. ROM is typically reduced with the greatest deficit found with dorsiflexion.

Disclosures: Dr M.E. Brage is a paid consultant and paid presenter for OsteoMed, and for Wright Medical Technology. Dr M.D. Johnson has nothing to disclose.
[a] Division of Orthopaedics, University of Alabama at Birmingham, 1313 13th Street South, Birmingham, AL 35205, USA; [b] Department of Orthopaedics, University of Washington, 1959 Northeast Pacific Street, Box 356500, Seattle, WA 98195, USA
* Corresponding author.
E-mail address: michaeljohnson@uabmc.edu

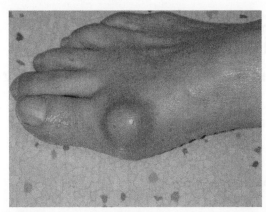

Fig. 1. Clinical appearance of foot with hallux rigidus with dorsal osteophyte that caused pain when donning shoes.

Radiographic evaluation may reveal joint space narrowing on the anteroposterior and oblique views. The lateral view may also show a dorsal osteophyte along with elevatus of the first metatarsal (MT). Elevatus of the MT is relative dorsiflexion of the MT in relationship to the proximal phalanx of the hallux (**Fig. 2**).

Grading systems are available for hallux rigidus with the Coughlin and Shurnas[1] system most commonly used. It takes into account both physical examination findings and radiographic findings (**Table 1**). A radiographic grading system is offered by Hattrup and Johnson[2]:

- Grade 1: well-preserved joint space with mild to moderate osteophytes
- Grade 2: reduced joint space with moderate osteophytes, sclerosis, and cysts
- Grade 3: complete loss of joint space, marked osteophytes, and subchondral cysts within the MT head

Treatment of hallux rigidus typically begins with conservative methods. Approximately half of patients are treated successfully with nonoperative treatments.[3] Options

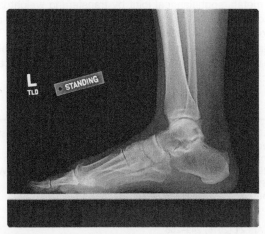

Fig. 2. Standing lateral radiograph shows both the dorsal osteophyte of the first MT as well as the elevatus of the first MT.

Table 1
Coughlin and Shurnas grading system for hallux rigidus

Grade	Range of Motion	Radiographs	Examination Findings
0	DF 40°–60° 10%–20% loss[a]	Normal	Stiffness and loss of passive ROM
1	DF 30°–40° 20%–50% loss	Dorsal spur, minimal joint narrowing	Mild, occasional pain at extremes of motion
2	DF 10°–30° 50%–75% loss	Dorsal + medial/lateral osteophytes <25% joint involvement on lateral radiograph Sesamoids normal	Moderate to severe pain; pain just before maximal dorsiflexion/plantarflexion
3	DF <10° 75%–100% loss PF loss of motion	Similar to grade 2 but >25% joint involvement Substantial joint narrowing and cysts Changes in the sesamoids	Constant pain and stiffness NO pain at mid-ROM
4	DF <10° 75%–100% loss PF loss of motion	Similar to grade 2 but >25% joint involvement Substantial joint narrowing and cysts Changes in the sesamoids	Constant pain and stiffness Pain at mid–ROM

Abbreviations: DF, dorsiflexion; PF, plantar flexion.
[a] Loss is in comparison to contralateral side.

include orthoses with a rigid shank under the hallux (Morton's extension), anti-inflammatories, intra-articular steroid injections, and activity and shoe modifications. Studies have shown that pain is reduced by intra-articular steroid and hyaluronate injections, but at 1 year, half of these patients elect for a surgical solution.[4] When conservative treatments fail, patients are offered surgical treatments. Surgical options include

- Cheilectomy
- Interpositional arthroplasty
- Osteotomies
- Fusion
- Arthroplasty
- Unipolar
  - MT
  - Phalangeal
- Bipolar

This article focuses on bipolar arthroplasty of the first metatarsophalangeal joint.

Arthroplasty of the great toe began in the 1950s with silicone implants similar to those used in the hands. These implants were designed essentially as a soft tissue spacer and could not bear the forces imparted by a weight-bearing joint. Consequently, they had a high failure rate due to reactive bone responses and implant fracture.[5] In an effort to obtain additional fixation and reduce silicone wear, double-stemmed silicone implants with grommets were introduced. These implants still had problems with silicone debris, foreign body reactions, osteolysis, and failure.[6,7] Patients reported fair subjective results with silicone implants, but enthusiasm waned after reports of systemic silicone complications, including silicone lyphadentitis,[8] brain cancer, and alopecia.[9]

Considering the success of metal on polyethylene implants in the hip and the knee, these materials began to be used in the first metatarsophalangeal joint. One of these early implants used a constrained polyethylene phalangeal component with a metal MT component. Results from this implant indicated that patients did not regain motion and experienced high rates of failure due to loosening.[10] The next generation of implants used either metal (titanium/cobalt-chrome [Co-Cr]) or ceramic components that were press fit with or without cement to anchor into the bone. Even with newer designs, there are still reported problems with subluxation and loosening.[11] Fourth-generation implants now use either threaded stems with a Morse taper or press-fit designs to secure the bearing surface.

Much of the difficulty with implant stability relates to the complicated biomechanics occurring at the first metatarsophalangeal joint. During normal gait, the center of rotation moves from a distal plantar position to a proximal dorsal position as the toe dorsiflexes. This transition begins as a rolling motion and then begins to slide with increasing dorsiflexion.[12–14] These complex biomechanics are demonstrated by the forces transmitted to the MT head that can exceed 120% body weight[15] and are doubled in high-heeled shoes.[16] These forces are even greater with arthroplasty components. Implant forces are higher because the prosthesis contact area is smaller than the native joint, thus generating higher pressures.[17]

Demand for pain relief along with preservation of motion has continued to drive innovation in implant designs. Studies are mixed regarding improvement of ROM after the replacement surgery.[18,19] Nonetheless, many patients are unwilling to undergo fusion due to the loss of motion for a multitude of reasons: desire to wear high-fashion shoes or to maintain the ability to squat and crouch for job requirements and for recreational pursuits. Gait studies have shown that patients with a fusion have a shorter stride length, less ankle plantar flexion at toe-off, and weaker push-off power.[20] These deficiencies may be preserved with arthroplasty due to normalization of load transfer across the forefoot.[21]

Currently, several bipolar implants are available in the United States. Most of the designs use titanium stems that are porous coated for press-fit or cemented implantation with a Co-Cr articulating surface on ultra–high-weight molecular polyethylene. **Table 2** shows images of bipolar implants currently available in the United States:

- Movement Great Toe (Integra, Plainsboro, New Jersey)
  - Three components are used—press-fit titanium stem with Co-Cr bearing surface on polyethylene.
  - Dorsal flange allows articulating surface during dorsiflexion and a plantar recess to allow for sesamoid excursion.
  - Suture holes in proximal phalanx allow for reattachment of plantar structures if necessary.
  - Phalangeal and MT components are fully interchangeable.
  - Bone is prepared via reaming over a guide wire. Cutting guide is used for dorsal MT cut.
- ToeMobile (Merete, New Windsor, New York)
  - Two components are used—cemented titanium stem with a Co-Cr bearing surface on polyethylene.
- ReFlexion (OsteoMed, Irving, Texas)
  - Three components are used—cemented titanium stem with a Co-Cr bearing surface on polyethylene.
  - MT stem is angulated to allow for intramedullary placement. MT bearing surface attaches to stem via Morse taper.

Table 2
Bipolar implants currently available in the United States

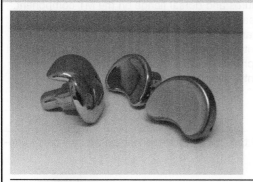	Movement Great Toe (Integra, Plainsboro, New Jersey)
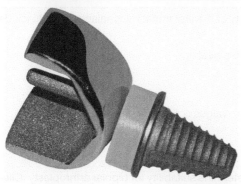	ToeMobile (Merete, New Windsor, New York)
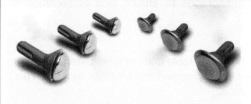	ReFlexion (OsteoMed, Irving, Texas)
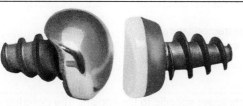	ToeMotion (Arthrosurface, Franklin Massachusetts)

- Bone is prepared with flat cuts on the MT and phalangeal sides, followed by alignment guides and power reamers.
- Phalangeal and MT components are fully interchangeable.
- ToeMotion (Arthrosurface, Franklin Massachusetts)

○ Three components are used: a titanium threaded stem with Morse taper and Co-Cr bearing surface on polyethylene.
○ There are dual implant curvatures and dorsal flange on the MT component.
○ Dorsal reamer is used to prepare dorsal MT.
- Futura (Tornier, Montbonnot, France)
  ○ There is 1 press-fit component—silicone with grommets.
- Swanson flexible (Wright, Memphis, TN)
  ○ There is 1 press-fit component—silicone with grommets.

INDICATIONS/CONTRAINDICATIONS
Indications

Indications for bipolar arthroplasty of the first metatarsophalangeal joint include end-stage degenerative arthritis.

Contraindications

Contraindications to bipolar arthroplasty of the first metatarsophalangeal joint include

- Current active infection
- Vascular disease precluding reliable healing
- Inflammatory arthrosis
- Hallux sesamoid arthritis
- Inadequate bone stock
- Advanced deformity; severe hallux valgus

SURGICAL TECHNIQUE/PROCEDURE
Preoperative Planning

Patient radiographs are assessed to determine suitability for bipolar arthroplasty. Clinical examination is correlated with radiographs to ensure lack of sesamoid-MT arthritis.

Preparation and Patient Positioning

Patients are placed prone on an operating room table and undergo general or regional anesthesia per surgeon preference. The leg is prepped in normal sterile fashion and a tourniquet is used per surgeon preference.

Surgical Approach

- Midline dorsal incision is used.
- The extensor hallucis longus is retracted laterally.
- The metatarsophalangeal joint capsule is elevated full thickness off of bone (**Fig. 3**).

Surgical Procedure

- The procedure should follow techniques specific to the implant. The description that follows is for the ReFlexion system.
- Any dorsal osteophytes are excised so as to create normal contour of distal MT (**Fig. 4**).
- A saw is used to excise 4-5 mm of the distal metatarsal. The blade is oriented to remove more bone dorsally versus plantarly.
- The saw is then used to excise 3-4 mm of bone from the phalangeal base. Care is taken to avoid the plantar plate with the bone cuts (**Fig. 5**).
- Any tear or rupture of the plantar plate must be repaired.

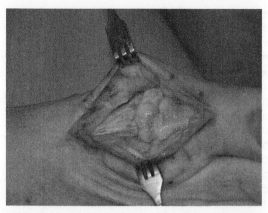

Fig. 3. Exposed dorsal metatarsophalangeal joint after dorsomedial approach.

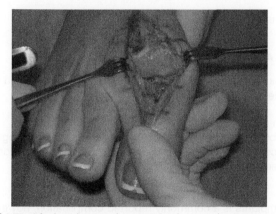

Fig. 4. The distal MT with dorsal osteophytes excised. Note the restoration of the normal contour of the distal MT.

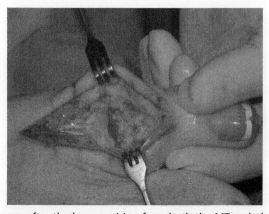

Fig. 5. The joint space after the bone excision from both the MT and phalangeal sides.

- The MT insertion point is identified.
- The metatarsal insertion point is midline with respect to the medial-lateral plane and just inferior to midline in the dorsal-plantar plane (**Fig. 6**)
- Careful insertion placement functions to minimize any elevation of the MT head
- Reaming is undertaken with the reamer rotated slightly laterally so that it is in line with the second MT.
- Phalangeal insertion point is centered medially-laterally and placed centrally from dorsal-plantar.
- Trials are inserted and ROM is examined (**Fig. 7**).
- Excessive shortening and over-lengthening are avoided.
- The MT stem is placed (**Fig. 8**).
- Phalangeal component is cemented into place.
- MT head is impacted onto Morse taper of MT stem (**Fig. 9**).
- Component position is verified with intraoperative imaging.
- The length of the hallux is assessed in relation to the previously placed mark on the second toe; 1 mm to 2 mm of shortening may aid in dorsiflexion and is preferred. Lengthening of the hallux is not well tolerated, however, and should be avoided.
- The wound is closed in layers

COMPLICATIONS AND MANAGEMENT

With modern designs, failure is usually by either infection or continued pain from loosening, subsidence, or fragmentation.[22]

Bone overgrowth or subsidence
   Although both bone overgrowth and subsidence are common radiographic findings, their presence does not always correlate with patient satisfaction and does not universally require removal.[23]

Loosening
   Loosening of implants is a commonly reported complication; however, it does not always correlate with patient satisfaction.[19,23,24]

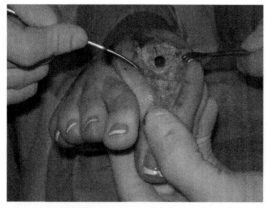

Fig. 6. The MT insertion point centered just inferior to midline.

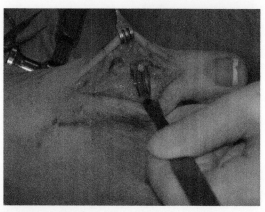

Fig. 7. The joint with trials in place.

Continued pain after first metatarsophalangeal arthroplasty

Pain typically stems from loosening, subsidence, or fragmentation, although loosening is not necessarily painful and careful evaluation is needed to determine the cause of pain after arthroplasty. Revision arthroplasty is an option, but bone loss at the first metatarsophalangeal joint and the lack of revision-specific implants preclude this option. These issues have led some investigators[22] to conclude that revision arthroplasty is never an option for failed first metatarsophalangeal joint arthroplasty.

Excision arthroplasty is another option after failed implant arthroplasty. Patients have been reported to have a 70% excellent outcome despite a trend toward cockup deformities and transfer metatarsalgia.[25] The patients best suited for excision arthroplasty may be those who were content with their arthroplasty despite radiographic appearance and who had an acute change in function.[22]

First metatarsophalangeal arthrodesis is the most commonly used operation for salvage of failed arthroplasty. Often with fusion after arthroplasty, the bony gap needs to be filled with structural interpositional graft.[26] One study[27] reporting on conversion from phalangeal hemiarthroplasty to fusion showed that visual analog

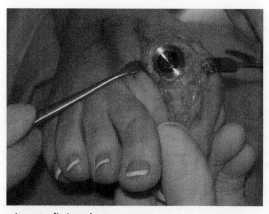

Fig. 8. The MT stem is press fit into bone.

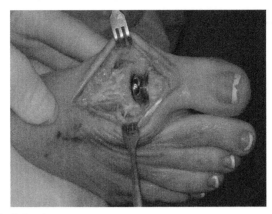

Fig. 9. Final implants in place.

scale (VAS) score improved from 7.8 to 0.75 and American Orthopaedic Foot & Ankle Society (AOFAS) score improvement from 36.2 to 85.3.[27] All patients achieved fusion; however, union took longer than a primary fusion. Fusion may be also indicated for a patient who was never satisfied with original arthroplasty results.[22]

Transfer metatarsalgia

Transfer metatarsalgia occurs due to excessive shortening of the first ray through the arthroplasty or instability leading to lateral forefoot overload. Evaluation should start with assessing for stability at the first metatarsophalangeal joint. If instability is present, it should be appropriately addressed based on the etiology. If the first ray is stable, the metatarsalgia may be addressed with standard interventions.

Infection

Deep infection is treated with a 2-stage revision. Stage 1 includes initial implant removal, cultures, antibiotic spacer, and a course of culture-specific antibiotics.[22] The second-stage reconstruction occurs after a minimum of 6 weeks and may involve structural bone graft.

Instability

Instability is an infrequent complication[28] and may be avoided with careful attention to implant sizing and soft tissue tensioning. It is critical to repair any plantar plate tears intraoperatively to avoid instability. If repair is not possible, fusion may be required to obtain adequate stability. Refractory instability of other causes is best treated with arthrodesis.

Sesamoid impingement and incarceration

Sesamoid impingement and incarceration occur when implants are undersized (**Fig. 10**). Incarceration is treated with revision arthroplasty with larger components or arthrodesis.

POSTOPERATIVE CARE

- Patient is placed into a sterile dressing that is left intact until follow-up.
- Immediate full weight bearing is allowed in a postoperative shoe.
- Sutures are removed approximately 14 days after surgery.

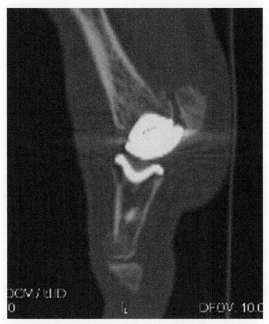

Fig. 10. Sagittal CT demonstrating incarceration of the sesamoids on an undersized implant.

- Physical therapy is ordered and Coban wrap is implemented for swelling reduction.

OUTCOMES

There is 1 randomized controlled trial comparing arthrodesis to 2-component arthroplasty (**Table 3**)[19]; 77 feet in 63 patients with hallux rigidus who had failed 12 months of conservative treatment were randomized to fusion using cerclage wire with Kirschner wire or 2-component unconstrained arthroplasty. Three fusions and 9 arthroplasties were lost to follow-up. Although these patients were not included in final data analysis, 6 of the 9 arthroplasty patients underwent a revision surgery. The remaining patients were followed for minimum of 24 months. The study is confounded by protocol deviation due to phalangeal loosening. After 18 months, 5 of the 30 arthroplasty patients complained of pain and had radiolucent lines around the phalangeal component with loosening. At this point, the investigators made the decision to change protocol and cement the phalangeal components for the remaining 9 patients. Overall, fusion patients had better outcomes in regards to pain, function, and alignment. There was no significant difference, however, in satisfaction between the groups.

A second study compared hemiarthroplasty to total arthroplasty to fusion and found no difference in outcome between hemiarthroplasty and total arthroplasty,[29] although arthrodesis had better outcomes than total arthroplasty or hemiarthroplasty.

Additional studies have suggested difficulty with return to sport after arthroplasty. Many patients had a decrease in sporting activity and had substantial difficulty returning to higher impact activities, such as soccer and running.[30]

Further study results may be seen in **Table 3**. Many of the studies are small series with relatively short follow-up. Additionally, the surgical indications vary from only

Table 3
Outcomes of bipolar arthroplasties

Authors, Year, Study Type, Country	Implant	Toes (Patients)	Follow-up (mo)	Outcomes	Revision Rate	Radiolucencies	Comments
Duncan et al,[31] 2014, retrospective, UK	ToeFit Plus (Plus Orthopedics, Switzerland)	69 (57)	22	AOFAS to 100 postoperative	8.7%	33.3%	All radiolucencies at the phalangeal component; nonprogressive in 19 (27.5%); intraoperative complications: 10% with either MT or phalangeal fx
Erkocak et al,[32] 2013, retrospective, Turkey	ToeFit Plus	26 (24)	29.9	AOFAS 42.7–88.5 Good/excellent 80.8% VAS 7.4–1.9 ROM from 25.9° to 53.8°	0	7.7%	Indication: HR; prolonged wound healing (1); MT fx (1); radiolucency (2)
Lange et al,[33] 2008, prospective	ToeFit Plus	80 (78)	56	Kitaoka score 85 ROM 38.6°	10.3%	—	Indications: HR, AVN, silastic and Keller revision; prolonged wound healing (2); osteolysis (23); arthrofibrosis (3)
Kundert & Zollinger-Kies,[28] 2005	ToeFit Plus	14 (14)	36	—	21%	NA	Complications 16.6%: dislocation (2), persistent pain (1), loss ROM (7)
Daniilidis et al,[30] 2010, prospective	ToeFit Plus	23 (23)	18	AOFAS 44–82.5 VAS 7–2 ROM 28.1° to 52.7° 82.6% satisfied	0	13% phalangeal	Indication: HR
Pulavarti et al,[34] 2005, retrospective, UK	Bio-Action (OsteoMed, Addison, Texas)	36 (32)	47	78% good/excellent 79% return to normal lifestyle 88% improvement in function Mean arc motion 44° Hallux metatarsophalangeal scale 26–78 Dorsiflexion from 5° to 45°	5.5%	33%	Indications: HR, HV, revision, RA; 33% loosening and subsidence, mostly MT; 1 intraoperative complication while inserting MT component

Study	Implant	N (pts)	Mean follow-up (mo)	Outcome	Complication	Loosening	Comments
Sinha et al,[35] 2010, retrospective, UK	Bio-action	14 (14)	61	AOFAS 62, 58% good excellent	14.3%	93.3% phalangeal 86.6% MT	Procedure abandoned due to poor objective results; universal signs of loosening did not correlate with subjective results
Olms & Dietze,[36] 1999, retrospective, Germany	Bio-action	21 (21)	24	17 less pain than before surgery, 77% good excellent, ROM 10° to 50°, 81% no pain	0	0	Indications: HR, failed resection arthroplasty, lack of toe purchase in 5 pts and metatarsalgia in 4 pts, 3 periarticular ossifications
Ess et al,[37] 2002, prospective, Finland	ReFlexion	10 (10)	24	60% good/excellent, AOFAS 41–84, VAS from 7.6 to 1.1, Dorsiflexion 25°	10%	NA	Indications: HR, malalignment (3), loosening (1); 1 reoperation due to recurrent HV
Fuhrmann et al,[38] 2003, prospective, Germany	ReFlexion	43 (41)	39	AOFAS from 51 to 74, VAS from 7.9 to 1.6, Dorsiflexion from 25° to 45°	9%	23% at phalangeal components 9% MT components	Indications: HR, revision arthroplasty, failed resection arthroplasty; 15 phalangeal components were cemented due to inadequacy of press fit; 5 additional were cemented on phalangeal and MT side; 60.5% radiologic or clinical malalignment
Gibson & Thomson,[19] 2005, prospective randomized controlled trial, UK	Biomet (Warsaw, Indiana)	39 (27)	24	VAS 6.0–2.7, ROM gain poor	15.4%	50%	Indication: HR tended to bear weight on outer border; 45% improvement at 2 y; 6/39 revised—phalangeal loosening; 40% would not undergo surgery again

(continued on next page)

Table 3
(continued)

Authors, Year, Study Type, Country	Implant	Toes (Patients)	Follow-up (mo)	Outcomes	Revision Rate	Radiolucencies	Comments
Koenig & Horwitz,[39] 1996, prospective, US	Biomet Total Toe	61 (59)	60	51 pts excellent 10 pts compromised result Koenig score 31.7–88	6.6%	NA	Indications: HR, HV, revision
Chee et al,[40] 2011, retrospective, UK	MOJE (Orthosonics Ltd., Edinburgh, Scotland)	41 (37)	33	92% satisfied 90% good/excellent AOFAS and HMPI Dorsiflexion from 9° to 15° Total ROM from 28° to 34°	7.3%	47.4% phalanx and 26.3% MT	Indications: HR 92% satisfied; no correlation between loosening and pts satisfaction; 19% would not have surgery again; 6 had loosening and 3 had subsidence of both components; 33% still taking analgesia medications
McGraw et al,[41] 2010, prospective, UK	MOJE	63 (48)	44	AOFAS from 56 to 72 Satisfaction score 7.6 67% minimal to no pain 91% implant survival 84% would have procedure again	7.9%	58% loosening	Indications: HR, failed fusions, and Keller; 57% MT and 56% phalangeal subsided; 58% loosening; subsidence associated with greater margin of uncovered bone under prosthesis
Barwick & Talkhani,[42] 2008, retrospective, UK	MOJE	24 (22)	26	63% very satisfied 20% dissatisfied AOFAS to 80 62.5% still with pain	12.5%	NA	Indications: HR, HV; excluded RA and revision silicones; 16% malaligned implants; 25% heterotopic ossification within the joint

Study	Implant	N (feet)		Outcome	Revision	Radiographic	Notes
Arbuthnot et al,[43] 2008, prospective, UK	MOJE	42 (40)	21	AOFAS 36–84.2 ROM 4.9° to 33.3° 82.5% satisfied	2.4%	13% (4/30 radiographs available)	ROM at final fu, <50% of what it was intraoperatively; only 10 pts had fu at 24 mo
Brewster et al,[44] 2010, prospective, UK	MOJE	32 (29)	34	AOFAS 74 40.6% good/excellent	6.25%	3.1% loosening	Indications: HR, failed Keller, and arthroplasty 18.75%; postoperative complications: 50% pts 30° ROM, 9% pts 75° ROM
Ibrahim & Taylor,[45] 2004, retrospective, UK	MOJE	11 (8)	17	Postoperative AOFAS 83 FFI 0	0 revision	NA	1 stress fx 2–3 MT, 1 dislocation, 1 exploration for pain
Omonbude & Faraj,[46] 2004, retrospective, UK	MOJE	14 (13)	12	AOFAS from 43 to 95 10 pts excellent ROM from 3.2° to 8.5°	7%	No specific comment	Audible squeaking noted
Nagy et al,[24] 2014, retrospective, UK	MOJE	31 (24)	81	AOFAS 72 FFI 27 45% poor	16%	52% 45% subsidence	Indications: HR and revision; satisfaction high (77%) despite poor (45%) clinical outcomes; implant survivorship 92% at 5 y, 85% at 7 y, 68% at 9 y; 36% with angular change of implant >10°

Abbreviations: AOFAS, AOFAS hindfoot score; AVN, avascular necrosis; FFI, foot function index; fu, follow-up; fx, fracture; HMPI, hallux metatarsal phalangeal-interphalangeal index; HR, hallux rigidus; HV, hallux valgus; pts, patients; RA, rheumatoid arthrtis.

hallux rigidus to hallux valgus, revision arthroplasty, and rheumatoid arthritis, confounding the interpretation of results.

SUMMARY

Total toe replacement of the first metatarsophalangeal joint is an evolving technology. Enthusiasm for implantation waned after early implants had substantial problems with loosening and osteolysis. Newer implants have adopted bearing surfaces and fixation principles similar to those used in hip and knee arthroplasty. These newer implants and techniques offer options to those patients seeking pain relief from hallux rigidus and are unwilling to accept the loss of motion associated with fusion. Well-controlled studies using these newer implants, however, are lacking and further research is needed to guide treatment decisions.

REFERENCES

1. Coughlin MJ, Shurnas PS. Hallux Rigidus. Grading and long term results of operative treatment. J Bone Joint Surg Am 2003;85-A(11):2072–88.
2. Hattrup SJ, Johnson KA. Subjective results of hallux rigidus following treatment with cheilectomy. Clin Orthop Relat Res 1988;226:182–91.
3. Grady JF, Axe TM, Zager EJ, et al. Retrospective analysis of 772 patients with hallux limitus. J Am Podiatr Med Assoc 2002;92:102–8.
4. Pons M, Alvarez F, Solana J, et al. Sodium hyaluronate in the treatment of hallux rigidus: a single-blind, randomized study. Foot Ankle Int 2007;28(1):38–42.
5. Granberry W, Noble P, Bishop J, et al. Use of a hinged silicone prosthesis for replacement arthroplasty of the first metatarsophalangeal joint. J Bone Joint Surg Am 1991;73:1453–9.
6. Cracchiolo AS, Swanson GD. The arthritic great toe metatarsophalangeal joint: a review of flexible silicone implant arthroplasty from two medical centers. Clin Orthop Relat Res 1981;(157):64–9.
7. Cracchiolo AS, Weltmer JB, Lian G, et al. Arthroplasty of the first metatarsophalangeal joint with a double-stem silicone implant. Results in patients who have degenerative joint disease failure of previous operations, or rheumatoid arthritis. J Bone Joint Surg Am 1992;74(4):552–63.
8. Lim WT, Landrum K, Weinberger B. Silicone lyphadenitis secondary to implan degeneration. J Foot Surg 1983;22:243–6.
9. Husson G, Herrinton LJ, Brox WT. A cohort study of systemic and local complications of toe prostheses. Am J Orthop (Belle Mead NJ) 2003;32(12):585–92.
10. Weil LS, Pollack RA, Goller WL. Total first joint replacement in hallux valgus and hallux rigidus. Long-term results in 484 cases. Clin Podiatry 1984;1(1):103–29.
11. Cook E, Cook J, Rosenblum B, et al. Meta-analysis of first metatarsophalangeal joint implant arthroplasty. J Foot Ankle Surg 2009;48(2):180–90.
12. Roukis TS, Jacobs PM, Dawson DM, et al. A prospective comparision of clinical, radographic, and intraoperative features of hallux rigidus. J Foot Surg 2002; 41(5):76–95.
13. Hetherington VJ, Carnett J, Patterson BA. Motion of the first metatarsophalangeal joint. J Foot Surg 1989;28(1):13–9.
14. Shereff MJ, Bejjani FJ, Kummer FJ. Kinematics of the metatarsophalangeal joint. J Bone Joint Surg Am 1986;68A(3):392–8.
15. Jacob HA. Forces acting in the forefoot during normal gait-an estimate. Clin Biomech 2001;16:783–92.

16. McBride ID, Wyss UP, Cooke TD, et al. First metatarsophalangeal joint reaction forces during high-heel gait. Foot Ankle 1991;11:282–8.

17. Schneider T, Dabirrahmani D, Gillies RM, et al. Biomechanical comparison of metatarsal head designs in first metatarsophalangeal joint arthroplasty. Foot Ankle Int 2013;34(6):881–9.

18. Maffulli N, Papalia R, Palumbo A, et al. Quantitative review of operative management of hallux rigidus. Br Med Bull 2011;98:75–98.

19. Gibson JN, Thomson CE. Arthrodesis or total replacement arthroplasty for hallux rigidus: a randomized controlled trial. Foot Ankle Int 2005;26:680–90.

20. DeFrino PF, Brodsky JW, Pollo FE, et al. First metatarsophalangeal arthrodesis: a clinical, pedobarographic and gait analysis study. Foot Ankle Int 2002;23(6):496–502.

21. Wetke E, Zerahn B, Kofed H. Prospective analysis of a first MTP total joint replacement. Evaluation by bone mineral densitometry, pedobarography, and visual analoge score for pain. Foot Ankle Surg 2012;18:136–40.

22. Greisberg J. The failed first metatarsophalangeal joint implant arthroplasty. Foot Ankle Clin 2014;19(3):343–8.

23. Kim PJ, Hatch D, Didomenico LA, et al. A multicenter retrospective review of outcomes for arthrodesis, hemi-metallic joint implant, and resectional arthroplasty in the surgical treatment of end-stage hallux rigidus. The J Foot Ankle Surg 2012;51(1):50–6.

24. Nagy MT, Walker CR, Sirikonda SP. Second-generation ceramic first metatarsophalangeal joint replacement for hallux rigidus. Foot Ankle Int 2014;35(7):690–8.

25. Kitaoka HB, Holiday AD, Chao EY, et al. Salvage of failed first metatarsophalangeal joint implant arthroplasty by implant removal and synovectomy: clinical and biomechanical evaluation. Foot Ankle Int 1992;13(5):243–50.

26. Gross CE, Hsu AR, Lin J, et al. Revision MTP arthrodesis for failed MTP arthroplasty. Foot & Ankle Specialist 2013;6(6):471–8.

27. Garras DN, Durinka JB, Bercik M, et al. Conversion arthrodesis for failed first metatarsophalangeal joint hemiarthroplasty. Foot Ankle Int 2013;34(9):1227–32.

28. Kundert HP, Zollinger-Kies H. Endoprosthetic replacement of hallux rigidus. Orthopade 2005;34(8):748–57.

29. Erdil M, Elmadag NM, Polat G, et al. Comparison of arthrodesis, resurfacing hemiarthroplasty, and total joint replacement in the treatment of advanced hallux rigidus. The J Foot Ankle Surg 2013;52(5):588–93.

30. Daniilidis K, Martinellie N, Marinozzi A. Recreational sport activity after total replacement of the first metatarsophalangeal joint: a prospective study. Int Orthop 2010;34(7):973–9.

31. Duncan NS, Farrar NG, Rajan RA. Early results of first metatarsophalangeal joint replacement using the ToeFit-Plus prosthesis. The J Foot Ankle Surg 2014;53(3):265–8.

32. Erkocak OF, Senaran H, Altan E, et al. Short-term functional outcomes of first metatarsophalangeal total joint replacement for hallux rigidus. Foot Ankle Int 2013;34(11):1569–79.

33. Lange J, Merk H, Barz T, et al. Titanium arthroplasty toe fit plus for the hallux metatarsophalangeal joint. Z Orthop Unfall 2008;146(5):609–15 [in German].

34. Pulavarti RS, McVie JL, Tulloch CJ. First metatarsophalangeal joint replacement using the bio-action great toe implant: intermediate results. Foot Ankle Int 2005;26(12):1033–7.

35. Sinha S, McNamara P, Bhatia M, et al. Survivorship of the bio-action metatarso-phalangeal joint arthroplasty for hallux rigidus: 5-year follow-up. Foot Ankle Surg 2010;16(1):25–7.

36. Olms K, Dietze A. Replacement arthroplasty for hallux rigidus. 21 patients with a 2-year follow-up. Int Orthop 1999;23:240–3.

37. Ess P, Hamalainen M, Leppilahti J. Non-constrained titanium-polyethylene total endoprosthesis in the treatment ofhallux rigidus. A prospective clinical 2-year follow-up study. Scand J Surg 2002;91(2):202–7.

38. Fuhrmann RA, Wagner A, Anders JO. First metatarsophalangeal joint replace-ment: the method of choice for end-stage hallux rigidus? Foot Ankle Clin 2003; 8:711–21, vi.

39. Koenig RD, Horwitz LD. The biomet total toe system utilizing the koenig score: a five-year review. The J Foot Ankle Surg 1996;35(1):23–6.

40. Chee YH, Clement N, Ahmed I, et al. Functional outcomes following ceramic total joint replacement for hallux rigidus. Foot Ankle Surg 2011;17(1):8–12.

41. McGraw IW, Jameson SS, Kumar CS. Mid-term results of the Moje Hallux MP joint replacement. Foot Ankle Int 2010;31(7):592–9.

42. Barwick TW, Talkhani IS. The MOJE total joint arthroplasty for 1st metatarsopha-langeal osteoarthritis: a short-term retrospective outcome study. Foot (Edinb) 2008;18:150–5.

43. Arbuthnot JE, Cheung G, Balain B, et al. Replacement arthroplasty of the first metatarsophalangeal joint using a ceramic-coated endoprosthesis for the treat-ment of hallux rigidus. The J Foot Ankle Surg 2008;47(6):500–4.

44. Brewster M, McArthur J, Mauffrey C, et al. Moje first metatarsophalangeal replacement–a case series with functional outcomes using the AOFAS-HMI score. The J Foot Ankle Surg 2010;49(1):37–42.

45. Ibrahim T, Taylor GJSC. The new press-fit ceramic Moje metatarsophalangeal joint replacement: short-term outcomes. Foot 2004;14(3):124–8.

46. Omonbude OD, Faraj AA. Early results of ceramic/ceramic fist metatarsophalan-geal joint replacement. Foot 2004;14(4):204–6.

Total Ankle Arthroplasty

An Overview of the Canadian Experience

Warren C.W. Latham, BScH, MD, FRCSC, Johnny T.C. Lau, MD, MSc, FRCSC*

KEYWORDS

- Total ankle arthroplasty • Salto • HINTEGRA • INBONE • Zimmer • Mobility

KEY POINTS

- Mobile-bearing total ankle arthroplasty use has decreased in favor of fixed-bearing implants in Canada.
- Ankle arthroplasty is still a technically demanding procedure despite improvement in ankle arthroplasty and design.
- Canadian intermediate-term outcome studies comparing ankle arthroplasty and ankle arthrodesis identify comparable clinical results.

INTRODUCTION

Although early results from total ankle arthroplasty (TAA) have demonstrated improved functional outcomes versus ankle arthrodesis,[1,2] complication rates with TAA insertion are still substantial and the procedure should be restricted to patients with valid operative criteria and surgeons with sufficient experience.[3] Since its inception in the 1970s, with each successive iteration or phase of TAA development has come the realization that deformity correction, soft tissue balancing, and patient education are all equally important to successful outcomes.[4]

TAA has two fundamental design concepts: fixed/constrained and mobile-bearing. Initial device designs were highly constrained, whereas second- and third-generation systems are cementless two- or three-component systems with a polyethylene insert mobile or incorporated into the tibial or talar component (fixed).[5] Early complications specific to all TAA include a potential risk for malleolar fracture secondary to bone resection from the tibia.[6] Wound complications are also an issue, although they decrease with increasing surgical experience.[3]

Multiple implant options are available in Canada including fixed- and mobile-bearing designs. Mobile-bearing implants have had Health Canada approval since 2001

Dr Latham has nothing to disclose. Dr Lau is a consultant for Bioaventus Canada, and is a consultant and receives royalties from Zimmer.
University of Toronto, Toronto, Ontario, Canada
* Corresponding author. University Health Network - Toronto Western Division, 399 Bathurst Street, 1 East Wing-438, Toronto, Ontario, M5T 2S8.
E-mail address: drjohnnylau@gmail.com

(Scandavian Total Ankle Replacement [STAR], Waldemar Link, Hamburg, Germany), and the HINTEGRA (Integra Lifesciences, Newdeal SA, Lyon, France) was approved in 2003. Fixed-bearing implant use has been increasing since 2009 with the approval of the INBONE system (Wright Medical Group, INBONE Technologies Inc, Boulder, CO) and the Zimmer trabecular metal total ankle replacement (TAR; Zimmer Biomet, Oakville, Ontario, Canada) in 2013.

INDICATIONS AND CONTRAINDICATIONS TO TOTAL ANKLE REPLACEMENT

TAR is indicated for degenerative joint disease of the tibiotalar joint caused by trauma, osteoarthritis, and rheumatoid arthritis.[7] Relative contraindications to TAR include osteoporosis, smoking, diabetes mellitus, immunosuppression, neurologic disease, vascular disease, age, severe malalignment, instability, and avascular necrosis (AVN) of the talus.[7] Absolute contraindications are active infection, Charcot neuro-arthropathy, and peripheral vascular disease (PVD).[7]

SURGICAL PLANNING

Surgical planning begins with a detailed history (Hx) and physical (Px) examination including the following[2]: muscle function, ankle range of motion (ROM), tendon excursion, standing limb alignment, gait, strength, peripheral vascular examination, skin quality, and hindfoot.

Next is a radiographic assessment with full-length limb alignment radiographs covering coronal plane malalignment and extra-articular malalignment. Computed tomography scan should include bone cyst evaluation, intra-articular pathology, and adjacent joint pathology. MRI is called for when there is concern regarding AVN. Finally, ischemic index evaluation is made.

SURGICAL APPROACH

All TAA models, except for the Zimmer implant, use a standard anterior approach to gain access to the tibiotalar joint.[8] The patient should be in supine position with a hip bump so that the coronal plane is parallel to the floor. A nonsterile tourniquet is used. A midline incision is centered one fingerbreadth lateral to the anterior tibial spine. The incision is started approximately 6 to 8 com proximal to the tibiotalar joint line and carried past the joint line by 4 to 5 cm.

Sharp dissection down through the skin and subcutaneous tissue, with ample care of the soft tissues, is followed by marking of the superficial peroneal nerve (SPN) nerve with a marking pen so it may be protected during the entirety of the case. The extensor retinaculum is incised in line with the skin incision and the interval between the extensor hallucis longus (EHL) and tibialis anterior (TA) tendons is identified.

An incision is made over the extensor hallucis longus (EHL) tendon sheath, and the neurovascular bundle is retracted laterally. The TA is maintained within its sheath to prevent postoperative bowstringing. Hemostasis is achieved with electrocautery. Self-retaining retractors are inserted to retract the lateral and medial soft tissues. Excessive ROM of the ankle should be avoided with self-retainers in situ to prevent damage to the skin edges.

The joint capsule is incised in line with the skin incision creating medial and lateral flaps via periosteal elevation. These flaps should be continued until both the medial and lateral gutters can be visualized. The elevation of the joint capsule is extended just to the level of the talonavicular joint. Anterior tibial and talar osteophytes are now excised. An osteotome may now be inserted to help determine rotation, varus/valgus malalignment, and instability of the joint.

The Zimmer TAA is in inserted through a lateral approach.[9] A lateral incision is made over the fibular ending distal to the fibular tip, protecting the SPN at the proximal extent. Anterior talofibular ligament (ATFL) and anterior inferior tibiofibular ligament (AITFL) are sectioned before an oblique fibular osteotomy is performed. Proximal fragment medial border should be 1 to 1.5 cm proximal to the tibiotalar joint line. Externally rotate the fibular fragment while incising the peroneal retinaculum and the posterior inferior tibiofibular ligament (PITFL). The fibula is then rotated down, and secured to the calcaneus with a k-wire. The medial portion of the joint is exposed via a standard anteromedial approach. As with an anterior approach all osteophytes are removed, and the posterior capsule is released.

All surgical approaches may require adjunctive procedures, including tendo Achilles lengthening or gastrocnemius release to ensure adequate dorsiflexion of the ankle before joint preparation.

THE MOBILITY TOTAL ANKLE REPLACEMENT
The Prosthesis

The Depuy Mobility TAR (Depuy International, Beeston and Holbeck Ward, United Kingdom) is an uncemented, third-generation mobile-bearing implant that has been commonly used in Europe and Canada (**Fig. 1**). The tibial component of the Mobility has a flat plate that provides posterior and anterior cortical support. The talar and tibial components are porous coated cobalt chrome, and the meniscal-bearing insert is ultra-high-molecular-weight polyethylene (UHMWPE). The tibial component has a

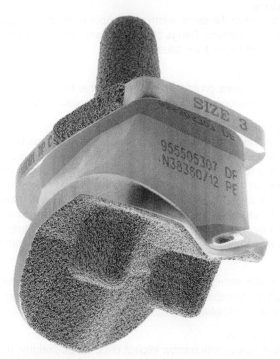

Fig. 1. Mobility total ankle prosthesis. (*Courtesy of* Depuy Synthes, Markham, ON; with permission.)

nonmodular intramedullary stem, whereas the talar component is cylindrical. The talar dome is press-fit into three prepared grooves within the talus, one central sulcus with two lateral fin grooves. The UHMWPE insert has fully congruent surfaces with both components making it semiconstrained. The polyethylene is narrower superiorly to prevent edge loading and reducing wear.[4]

In a Canadian study published in 2013, Daniels and colleagues[10] looked at 88 Mobility TAAs implanted in 85 patients, with the most common underlying diagnosis being post-traumatic arthritis (53%). Patients were reviewed at regular intervals postoperatively, with clinical and radiographic assessment. The mean follow-up time was 40 months (range, 30–60 months). Bone-implant interface abnormalities were identified in 33 ankles with a retained prostheses (43%). Thirty (91%) of these involved zones around the tibial plate. In total, eight TAAs required revision. The cumulative survival was 89.6% (95% confidence interval [CI], 80.8–94.8) at 3 years and 88.4% (95% CI, 79.3–93.9) at 4 years. Early results of the Mobility TAA for independent researchers do not match those reported by other surgeons. High rates of bone-implant interface abnormalities around the tibial plate are concerning but require longer follow-up to determine their clinical significance. This study led to decreased use of the Mobility implant across Canada.

Surgical Technique

External tibial alignment guide
Parallel to the long axis of the tibia, mandatory to have full length mechanical axis views.[9]

Tibial plafond resection
Oscillating saw for vertical cut, avoid extending cut into the medial malleolus.

Talar and tibial sizing
Sizes 1 to 6, guides have the same width as components, always downsize if size in doubt to prevent impingement. Gauge should be centered over talus, frequently tibial component is one size larger than talus.

Tibial window resection
Determines medial to lateral prosthesis positioning, the tibial component position depends on the talar component. Use thinnest available saw blade for tibial resection.

Superior talar flat cut resection
Talar jig is to be inserted with the foot at 90°. There are four sizes to jig based on estimated bearing thickness. When pinning the jig to talus varus/valgus position reduction can be manual. Insertion of the talar center guide shows the center of the anteroposterior (AP) position on the talar dome. Arthritic ankles may be translated anteriorly, in which case the talar center guide is advanced anteriorly the same amount. Posterior talar cutting blocks are available in two sizes (1–4, or 5/6). The anterior chamfer mill and guide require increase stability with externally manual pressure. After removing the anterior talar milling guide a rongeur is used to trim any bony prominences.

Trial insertion
Ensure that talar trial is sitting flush. If not then check for talar bony impingement, and talar sulcus and fin slots preparation. Ensure there is no talar overhang. Check for tibial trial impingement on the fibula.

Final component insertion
Talar component is seated with narrow aspect directed posteriorly. Axially distraction is required to insert the tibial component. Resected anterior bone window is reinserted after removing bone the width of tibial stem.

Rippstein and coworkers[11] detailed the early results of 200 Mobility TARs in 2008. One hundred consecutively performed TARs from the Schultess Clinic and 100 from Wrightington Hospital, Wigan were evaluated. The follow-up was at an average of 36 months (range, 24–50). In 20% of the cases, a gastrosoleus lengthening was performed, and 8% of cases underwent other adjunct procedures. Complications included intraoperative malleolar fractures (6%), delayed wound healing (4%), and late medial malleolar fractures (2%). One early infection occurred. Revision to an arthrodesis or a change of either component was required in five patients because of aseptic loosening. A technical error in one patient led to subluxation of the insert.

Wood and colleagues[12] published early results from their prospective study that included 100 Mobility implants performed in 96 patients between 2003 and 2005. At a minimum follow-up of 5 years, a total of five ankles (5%) had to undergo revision surgery (two ankle fusions and three revision arthroplasties) resulting in 3- and 4-year survivorship of 97% (95% CI, 91%–99%) and 93.6% (95% CI, 84.7%–97.4%), respectively. In 14 ankles a radiolucent line or osteolytic cavity was observed. However, only in five ankles was it more than 10 mm in width. The authors presented encouraging short-term results that are comparable with those obtained using other modern three-component prostheses.

THE HINTEGRA TOTAL ANKLE PROSTHESIS
The Prosthesis

The HINTEGRA TAR has been used since 2000 in Europe and since 2003 in Canada (**Fig. 2**). This prosthesis is a third-generation implant that provides inversion-eversion stability through a unique design. Because the distal tibia metaphyseal cancellous

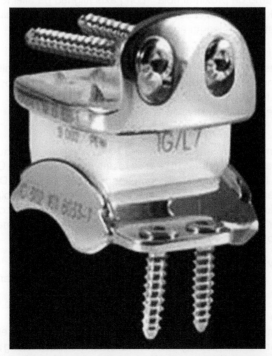

Fig. 2. HINTEGRA prosthesis. (*Courtesy of* Integra Lifesciences, Burlington, ON; with permission.)

bone has been associated with poor quality more than a few millimeters proximal to the joint, an important element in the rationale of the HINTEGRA prosthesis design was minimal tibial bone resection.[13]

It consists of a flat tibial component, a polyethylene inlay, and a convex conical talar component with a smaller medial radius. Both the tibial and talar components use shields for screw fixation. However, screw fixation was required to compensate for the lack of stems (Mobility) or anchorage bars (STAR prosthesis). In the early postoperative phase, before bone ingrowth provides adequate stability, loosening of the screws could be possible. Unique about this prosthesis is the anterior tibial flange to reduce postoperative heterotopic ossification and soft tissue adherence.[13] The prosthesis design also supports the use of revision components. The revision tibial tray is 8 to 12 mm thick rather than the standard 4-mm tray, and the talar revision component has a flat undersurface and two pegs to maximize contact in deficient bone stock and is double coated with a hydroxyapatite and titanium layer.[14]

The mobile-bearing polyethylene insert provides axial rotation and flexion-extension. The tibial component has peaks on the flat surface and the anterior phalange with screw hole fixation. The tibial component is flat with a 5° posterior inclination angle approximating the normal distal tibial surface. The anterior shield of the tibial component is designed to minimize stress shielding, and the medial and lateral rims of the talar component stabilize the insert. The talar component also has screw holes, and the radius is smaller medially than laterally. Much like the Mobility TAA, the superior surface of the polyethylene insert is smaller to prevent tibial impingement.[13]

Surgical Technique

Tibial jig placement
Placed using a clamp on proximal tibia.[9] Long axis aligned parallel to the tibia. Blunt osteotomes in ankle gutters to ensure appropriate rotation and centralization of the jig. Jig allows for rotation and length adjustments.

Distal tibial cut
Distal tibial cut has a 5° slope. In the presence of any bone loss, the distal tibial resection can be minimized. Avoid posterior medial structures. Use fluoroscopy to ensure tibial cut is flat. Medial cut is completed with reciprocating saw. Posterior bone must be completely removed to allow dorsiflexion.

Talar cut
A fibular osteotomy and/or a gastrocnemius recession may be required to correct equinus to allow talus to compress to talar jig to ensure a uniform cut. Cut may be deficient medial and lateral and must be completed after jig removal. Downsizing talar component can lead to less gutter impingement. Once talar jig is in place it is difficult to make small adjustments to translation and rotation. Posterior talar cut is performed with foot in planar flexion. A reciprocating saw is used to complete medial and lateral gutter cuts to 2 to 3 mm.

Ligament stability assessment
Green spacer (8 mm) is inserted into the joint to assess ROM and ligamentous instability.

Talus preparation
Jig needs to be impacted onto bone. Cuts may need to be revised to ensure complete apposition. Confirm on fluoroscopy correct station of the talus on long axis of the tibia. A trial spacer may now be placed.

Final component selection

Talar component is placed first, tibial component second. Hard tibial bone may prevent proper seating of pyramidal fixation pins. Ankle balancing can be completed with the trial polyethylene (PE) in place. Varus and valgus malalignment can be addressed using the HINTEGRA prosthesis.

In 2004, Hintermann and colleagues[15] described their experience with 122 HINTEGRA TAR. Of 122 TARs, eight had to be revised (four because of aseptic loosening of at least one component, one because of dislocation of the insert, and three for other complications). They reported that 84% of the TARs were satisfied. American Orthopaedic Foot and Ankle Society (AOFAS) scores improved from 40 points preoperatively to 85 points postoperatively. Eighty ankles (63%) were completely pain-free. Radiographically, migration of the talar component was noted in two ankles with no tibial components showing any signs of loosening (mean follow-up, 18.9 months).

Barg and colleagues[16] published a HINTEGRA TAA survivorship analysis in 684 patients in 2013. A total of 779 primary TAAs (741 patients) were performed between May 2000 and July 2010 with use of the HINTEGRA three-component prosthesis. The mean time to final follow-up (and standard deviation) was 6.3 ± 2.9 years. The overall survival rates were 94% and 84% after 5 and 10 years, respectively. Sixty-one ankles had a revision arthroplasty (27 both components, 13 the tibial component only, and 14 the talar component only) or were converted to a fusion.

Hintermann and colleagues[14] in 2013 reviewed a case series of 117 revision TARs using the HINTEGRA prosthesis. The estimated survival of the revision arthroplasties at 9 years was 83%, which compared favorably with the midterm results of primary arthroplasty.

INBONE TOTAL ANKLE ARTHROPLASTY
The Prosthesis

This implant uses unique intramedullary alignment instrumentation, combined with modular titanium tibial and talar stems (**Fig. 3**). This creates the theoretic advantage of better fixation in osteoporotic tibial bone and the possibility of subtalar fusion via the implant for revision cases.[17] Longer talar stems (48–66 mm) although not approved by the Food and Drug Administration are used when no subtalar motion exists, when there is substantial talar bone loss, or when subtalar fusion is planned as part of initial procedure.[18]

The INBONE TAR uses a specially designed foot-holding targeting device allowing for precise positioning of the components using fluoroscopic imaging. The tibial stem is a modular design with segments (12–18 mm in diameter), which is assembled within the resected ankle joint and then passed up into the tibia before being connected to the tibial baseplate.[9] The fundamental design concept is that of offloading the tibial and talar components with large stems. The talar dome with its double saddle design is two times larger than other Food and Drug Administration–approved TAR talar dome components.[4] The modularity of the implants, stems, differing polyethylene thicknesses, flat cut approach to the talus, and the optional use of longer calcaneal stems offer the possibility of revising other ankles to INBONE.[17]

The PROPHECY INBONE total ankle system uses preoperative imaging to create individualized cutting jigs for each patient.[9] Developed by Wright Medical for total knee arthroplasty, the PROPHECY uses computed tomography to create patient-specific ankle alignment guides to precisely size, place, and align the INBONE TAA components during surgery. All preoperative implant position decisions are integrated into the design of the patient-specific surface match alignment, thus reducing the surgical steps allowing for decreased operative time.

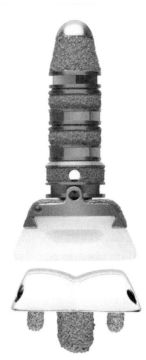

Fig. 3. INBONE prosthesis. (Image provided courtesy of Wright Medical Technology, Inc., Oakville, ON; with permission.)

In 2014, DeOrio and colleagues[19] published a case series of their early to mid-term results using the INBONE prosthesis. They identified 194 primary INBONE TAAs with a mean clinical follow-up of 3.7 years (range, 2.2–5.5 years). Patients demonstrated a significant improvement ($P<.003$) in visual analog scale (VAS) pain, American Orthopedic Foot and Ankle Surgeons (AOFAS), short musculoskeletal functional assessment (SMFA), and Short Form-36 (SF-36) scores at the time of final follow-up, compared with preoperative values, and in walking speed, sit to stand (STS) time, timed up and go (TUG) time, and four square step test (4SST) time at 2 years postoperatively, compared with preoperatively.

The mean coronal tibiotalar angle for varus and valgus ankles significantly improved postoperatively and was maintained until the time of final follow-up. The prevalence of unstable subsidence leading to impending failure was 5%, and the prevalence of revision was 6%. They authors concluded that patients undergoing TAA with the INBONE TAR demonstrated significant improvement in radiographic, functional, and patient-reported outcome scores at a mean of 3.7 years postoperatively, and the overall implant survival rate was 89%.

Surgical Technique

Intramedullary alignment

Heel must rest flat on leg holder frame footplate to ensure that the talar cut is not sloped posteriorly.[9] Foot holder must be perfectly parallel to the beam of the fluoroscope, one method to create a perfect mortise view. The fins of the guide rods must be centered on orthogonal fluoroscopic views. A 6-mm drill is inserted plantarly after soft tissue dissection to plantar calcaneal bone is carried out. Peck drilling is recommended to minimize skiving. The drill bit is advanced 8 cm into the tibia.

Bone cuts

Anterior cutting guide orientation and size is judged fluoroscopically. The guide should be place as close as possible to the joint without causing soft tissue compromise. Minimal medial malleolar resection is required. During excision the anterior tibial plafond is removed followed by the excised talar dome. Then the remaining tibial plafond is resected.

Tibial stem preparation

Tibial reaming is accomplished through plantar entry. Correct size reamer tip is inserted through the joint space and is screwed onto reamer driver. Reamer size is usually one size smaller that tibial base stem. Extract the reamer tip while reaming clockwise. A standard or long tibial tray baseplate is then trialed.

Talar component preparation

Talar trial is placed after thorough gutter debridement. No medial or lateral overhang should be present. Placing the ankle in a plantar flexed position, the talar trial is pinned in place. For INBONE II, 4-mm pegs are drilled. Talar stem reamer is used once the trial is removed.

Component implantation

Top two stem pieces (including tapered stem piece) are inserted simultaneously in the joint and placed in position by a plantarly inserted screwdriver. Sequential pieces are then inserted into the joint and connected with the xdrive screwdriver. Tibial baseplate is inserted last with Morse taper handle in line with antirotation notch. The tibial tray is then impacted onto the tibial stem via strike rod and mallet. Cement may be added to the nonarticular surface of the tibial tray before the tibial construct is terminally impacted. The talar component has 10- and 14-mm stems. The 10-mm stem is inserted on the back table and the 14-mm stem is impacted in position. Talar dome insert is then impacted with talar strike tool with the foot in plantar flexion. PE thickness can then be trialed and installed using a specific PE insert tool.

SALTO TOTAL ANKLE ARTHROPLASTY
The Prosthesis

The Salto-Talaris (Wright Medical Group, Memphis, Tennesee) TAA system design is a fixed-bearing modification of the Salto TAA (**Fig. 4**).[4] On the tibial side of the Salto-Talaris ankle the design requires fixed insertion of the UHMWPE liner. It is easily replaceable. The tibial side is fixed in the tibia by a pedestal attached to the tibial implant by a thin shaft. This pedestal is inserted into the tibia through a small cortical window. Although the central pedestal and instrumentation of the Salto-Talaris ankle arthroplasty system are designed to allow the trial tibia to rotate or "find" the correct position as determined by the talus the clinical application is more demanding and often little rotation occurs.[20]

The Salto total ankle prosthesis is a third-generation, cementless mobile-bearing three-component design developed in France.[21] The tibial component has a flat surface that faces the mobile-bearing, allowing free translation and rotation. The 3-mm medial rim is designed to avoid insert impingement against the medial malleolus, and the fixation peg and keel provide stability. The tibial component that comes into contact with the tibia seems to be the same as the Salto-Talaris TAR.[4]

The specific shape of the talar component mimics the natural talar geometry: the anterior width is wider than the posterior width and the lateral flange has a larger curvature radius than the medial. The mobile-bearing is manufactured from UHMWPE

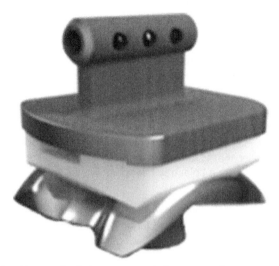

Fig. 4. Salto total ankle prosthesis (Image provided courtesy of Wright Medical Technology, Inc., Oakville, ON; with permission.)

and has full congruency with the talar component in flexion and extension and allows as much as 4° of varus and valgus movement in the coronal plane.[20]

The first clinical study on the Salto prosthesis was published in 2004. Bonnin and colleagues[22] implanted 98 consecutive Salto prostheses between 1997 and 2000. Ninety-three implants in 91 patients were reviewed clinically and radiographically at a mean follow-up of 35 months. Most patients were pain free and showed a significant functional improvement as assessed by AOFAS score (from 32.2 to 83.1 points). Two prostheses had to be converted to ankle fusion, resulting in survivorship of more than 95% at 68 months.

Bonnin and colleagues[21] have also presented survivorship analysis at 7 to 11 years in a retrospective review of 98 TARs. Six SALTO TARs had to be converted to ankle fusion and an additional 18 ankles underwent reoperation without ankle fusion (10-year survivorship, 65%; 95% CI, 50%–80%). The most common complications requiring additional surgery were bone cysts (11 ankles), fracture of polyethylene (five ankles), and nonspecific pain (three ankles).

Surgical Technique

Tibial alignment
The tibial extramedullary alignment guide is aligned parallel with anterior tibial crest in the coronal plane.[9] Coronal plane deformity can be corrected by shifting the guide medially or laterally. Osteotomes are placed in the medial and lateral gutters to use as goalposts to assess rotation. Resection level should aim to restore anatomic joint line.

Tibial cutting block
Appropriate-sized distal tibial cutting block is selected based on fluoroscopic imaging. Pins in the medial and lateral holes of the cutting block protect the malleoli from the oscillating saw.

Distal tibial resection
Cutting block is removed after distal tibial cut, and a reciprocating saw is used to connect medial and lateral drill holes. The distal tibial plafond is resected.

Talar preparation
Talar pin guide is attached to tibial alignment guide. Ankle is dorsiflexed to 5°. A reference pin is placed at the neck/body junction of the talus. Medial and lateral laminar spreaders are equally distracted. Fluoroscopy is used to assess the level of the talar cut after pin insertion; the cut should be flush to the pins.

Anterior talar chamfer
Apex of the anterior chamfer guide is placed on the apex of the talar resection. The talar position spacer is added to this guide for depth estimation. Rotation can be set using axis of the second toe. A milling device is used to complete the anterior chamfer cut.

Lateral chamfer cut/talar stem preparation
Align the handle of the lateral chamfer cutting guide with lateral talar cortical body and the second metatarsal. This guide allows for talar stem recession, and lateral chamfer preparation.

Insertion of trial components
Avoid medial overhang with talar trial. Next insert the trial tibia and PE insert. Ankle must be placed through ROM to allow tibial assembly to find ideal position. Now drilling for tibial keel can be completed. Keel cuts are rounded and connected using a reciprocating saw. Tibial trial is then replaced with PE inserts to assess ankle stability.

Insertion of implants
Talus is placed first and impacted, tibial and PE components second. Caudal pressure is applied on the heel to ensure that the tibial component remains flush with the tibia. Autograft is inserted into the tibial window.

ZIMMER TRABECULAR METAL TOTAL ANKLE ARTHROPLASTY
The Prosthesis

The Zimmer TAA implant has several unique design features (**Fig. 5**). Insertion of the implant is accomplished via a lateral approach using a rigid alignment frame and cutting assembly. An extensile lateral approach may reduce wound healing issues. The lateral approach creates the possibility of milling the distal tibia and talar dome surfaces, which allows the insertion of curved implants to follow the natural contour of the bony surfaces of the tibiotalar joint. A transfibular approach may also decrease the risk of injury to the neurovascular structures because anterior to posterior sawing is limited.[9]

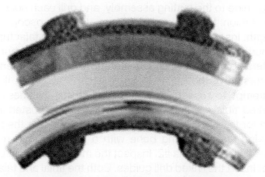

Fig. 5. Zimmer prosthesis. (Image provided courtesy of Wright Medical Group, Memphis, TN; with permission.)

The device is semiconstrained consisting of two components. The talar component is composed of trabecular metal and cobalt chromium with an intervening titanium layer. The high-density cross-linked tibial polyethylene tray is locked into the titanium surface of the tibial housing, and has a central ridge to correspond to the sulcus between the talar condyles. The Zimmer ankle features a three-fold fixation strategy: (1) coronally oriented tibial component rails, (2) trabecular metal (TM)–bone surface interface, and (3) small amounts of bone cement along the course of its four rails.[9]

Surgical Technique (See Lateral Approach)

Medial-lateral sizing

Place the sizer between the talus and tibial plafond abutting the articular portion of the medial malleolus.[9] If the size is in between two sizes, downsize to smaller tibial size. The tibial and talar sizes must match, and mismatch between tibial and talar sizes is not possible.

Frame assembly

Lateral ankle view must not be obscured by alignment rods and the anterior tibial crest is parallel to the longitudinal frame rods. Tibial tubercle should be oriented vertically. Perfect mortise view should be present on AP radiographs. Foot brackets are secured to the foot with tensor bandages at the level of the metatarsalphalangeal (MTP) joints. Calcaneal transfixation pin is placed 2.5 cm anterior to insertion of the Achilles. Talar pin is inserted into the talar neck, and must be inserted to avoid obscuring the lateral talus radiograph. Intra-articular joint deformity correction is performed using a laminar spreader. Tibial pins are inserted once deformity correction has been confirmed in all planes. Carbon bars may be used medially and anterior to create additional frame stability.

Anteroposterior sizing

Round down to avoid excessive overhang. AP size and medial-lateral (ML) size should match.

Positioning

Lateral cutting assembly locked in place. Standard cuts are 2 mm above the talar dome arc. Probe tracing should intersect talar articulation at its apex. Use cutting jigs marked "talus" and "tibia" to template bone cuts. Allows for fluoroscopic and direct visualization of coronal orientation of the new joint line.

Bone preparation

Secure the cutting guide to the cutting assembly, and drill each hole over the tibia and talus in a pecking fashion. Minimize drill deflection. Use fluoroscopy-guided drilling to ensure correct depth. Insert the burr into the burr guard using talar trial as a burr guard stop to prevent burring into the medial malleolus. Irrigate while burring. Peck drill a nest of tunnels lateral to medial through the anterior and then posterior talus. Anterior and posterior excursion of the burr can be limited by adjusting the corresponding stops. Do not attempt to resect talus through one full-thickness arc. Insert burr through hole marked tibia #1, and reset the anterior and posterior excursions. No spacer is required for the tibial burring. Again tibial drilling with the peck-drilling nest technique. Removing any remaining bone with a rongeur, then repeat the cutting sequence using the jig marked tibia #2. Inspect the medial gutter to remove any debris or impinging bone. Insert the linked drill guides. Both the tibial and talar should be flush to bone, and perpendicular to frame rods before creating sagittal rails for implant insertion. A rail hole stabilizer should be used after each rail hole is drilled.

Trialing

Three sizes of tibial provisional implants correspond to three available polyethylene inserts, which increase in 2-mm increments. K-wire is removed to allow fibular reduction and check for lateral impingement. Carbon fiber rods across the ankle joint are removed. Footplate support is removed. Valgus stability can now be assessed. Valgus laxity may be improved by retrialing with larger tibial provisional implant.

Implant insertion

Insertion of tibial provisional implant facilitates real talar component insertion. Gentle impaction is required once the path of the rail has been engaged. The polyethylene insert is attached to the tibial tray before insertion. Insert the tibial implant with ankle in mild plantar flexion then dorsiflex the ankle to apply compressive forces. Avoid vigorous impaction. Bone cement can be injected into each rail hole on the tibia and talus.

Repair and closure

Assess lateral joint congruency after fibular reduction and varus ankle stability. The fibula may now be adjusted to restore the mortise or adjust ligament tension. Fibular fixation is achieved with lateral plating. Transsyndesmotic fixation can be applied for a positive external rotation squeeze test. Repair the released ATFL.

COMPARATIVE STUDIES

In 2014, the Canadian Orthopaedic Foot and Ankle Society published intermediate term results comparing outcomes of TAA with ankle arthrodesis.[1] This prospective study evaluated intermediate-term outcomes of ankle replacement and arthrodesis in a large cohort at multiple centers, with variability in ankle arthritis type, prosthesis type, surgeon, and surgical technique.

Patients in the Canadian Orthopaedic Foot and Ankle Society Prospective Ankle Reconstruction Database were treated with TAR (involving Agility, STAR, Mobility, or HINTEGRA prostheses) or ankle arthrodesis by six subspecialty trained orthopedic surgeons at four centers between 2001 and 2007.

Data collection included demographics, comorbidities, and the Ankle Osteoarthritis Scale (AOS) and SF-36 scores. The preoperative and latest follow-up scores for patients with at least 4 years of follow-up were analyzed.

Of the 388 ankles (281 in the ankle replacement group and 107 in the arthrodesis group), 321 (83%; 232 ankle replacements and 89 arthrodeses) were reviewed at a mean follow-up of 5.5 ± 1.2 years. Patients treated with arthrodesis were younger, more likely to have diabetes, less likely to have inflammatory arthritis, and more likely to be smokers. Seven (7%) of the arthrodeses and 48 (17%) of the ankle replacements underwent revision. The major complications rate was 7% for arthrodesis and 19% for ankle replacement.

The AOS total, pain, and disability scores and SF-36 physical component summary score improved between the preoperative and final follow-up time points in both groups. The mean AOS total score improved from 53.4 points preoperatively to 33.6 points at the time of follow-up in the arthrodesis group and from 51.9 to 26.4 points in the ankle replacement group. Differences in AOS and SF-36 scores between the arthrodesis and ankle replacement groups at follow-up were minimal after adjustment for baseline characteristics and surgeon.

Intermediate-term clinical outcomes of TAR and ankle arthrodesis were comparable in a diverse cohort in which treatment was tailored to patient presentation; rates of reoperation and major complications were higher after ankle replacement.

In Canada multiple different ankle arthroplasty systems are readily available for use. The procedure itself continues to be technically demanding and require surgical sophistication and expertise. The Canadian Foot and Ankle Society continues to collect data to analyze outcomes of the total arthroplasty experience across the country.

COMPLICATIONS AND MANAGEMENT

Possible complications and their management are as follows[3,6]:

- Aseptic loosening or subsidence
  - More common in first- and second-generation implants
  - Rockering of the prosthesis
- Implant instability
  - Subluxation/ligament imbalance
  - Posttraumatic osteoarthritis
- Septic loosening
  - Early wound closure for postoperative wound problems
  - Careful handling of soft tissues is key
  - Avoid tight dressings, minimize tourniquet time
  - Two-stage revision required for deep infections
- Periprosthetic fracture
  - Iatrogenic, stress, traumatic
  - Intraoperative, early postoperative, late postoperative
  - Medial malleolus more common
- Pathologic wear
  - PE wear leads to periprosthetic osteolysis
  - Cyst formation: newer observed phenomena
  - Cysts more prevalent on the talar side
- Implant breakage
  - Rare
- Gutter impingement
  - Still a technically demanding procedure
  - Commonest reason for revision
  - Downsizing talar components
  - Adequate gutter resection
  - Single-photon emission computed tomography useful for diagnosis

REFERENCES

1. Daniels TR, Younger AS, Penner M, et al. Intermediate-term results of total ankle replacement and ankle arthrodesis: a COFAS multicenter study. J Bone Joint Surg Am 2014;96(2):135–42.
2. Bonasia DE, Dettoni F, Femino JE, et al. Total ankle replacement: why, when and how? Iowa Orthop J 2010;30:119–30.
3. Myerson MS, Mroczek K. Perioperative complications of total ankle arthroplasty. Foot Ankle Int 2003;24(1):17–21.
4. Cracchiolo A 3rd, Deorio JK. Design features of current total ankle replacements: implants and instrumentation. J Am Acad Orthop Surg 2008;16(9):530–40.
5. Gougoulias N, Khanna A, Maffulli N. How successful are current ankle replacements? A systematic review of the literature. Clin Orthop Relat Res 2010; 468(1):199–208.

6. McGarvey WC, Clanton TO, Lunz D. Malleolar fracture after total ankle arthroplasty: a comparison of two designs. Clin Orthop Relat Res 2004;(424):104–10.
7. Chou LB, Coughlin MT, Hansen S Jr, et al. Osteoarthritis of the ankle: the role of arthroplasty. J Am Acad Orthop Surg 2008;16(5):249–59.
8. Smith TW, Stephens M. Ankle arthroplasty. Foot Ankle Surg 2010;16(2):53.
9. Myers SH, Schon LC. 1st edition. Total ankle replacement: an operative manual, vol. 1. Baltimore (MD): Lippincoot Williams and Wilkins; 2014. p. 67–91.
10. Sproule JA, Chin T, Amin A, et al. Clinical and radiographic outcomes of the Mobility total ankle arthroplasty system: early results from a prospective multicenter study. Foot Ankle Int 2013;34(4):491–7.
11. Rippstein PF, Huber M, Coetzee JC, et al. Total ankle replacement with use of a new three-component implant. J Bone Joint Surg Am 2011;93(15):1426–35.
12. Wood PL, Karski MT, Watmough P. Total ankle replacement: the results of 100 Mobility total ankle replacements. J Bone Joint Surg Br 2010;92(7):958–62.
13. Barg A, Knupp M, Henninger HB, et al. Total ankle replacement using HINTEGRA, an unconstrained, three-component system: surgical technique and pitfalls. Foot Ankle Clin 2012;17(4):607–35.
14. Hintermann B, Zwicky L, Knupp M, et al. HINTEGRA revision arthroplasty for failed total ankle prostheses. J Bone Joint Surg Am 2013;95(13):1166–74.
15. Hintermann B, Valderrabano V, Dereymaeker G, et al. The HINTEGRA ankle: rationale and short-term results of 122 consecutive ankles. Clin Orthop Relat Res 2004;(424):57–68.
16. Barg A, Zwicky L, Knupp M, et al. HINTEGRA total ankle replacement: survivorship analysis in 684 patients. J Bone Joint Surg Am 2013;95(13):1175–83.
17. DeOrio JK. Revision INBONE total ankle replacement. Clin Podiatr Med Surg 2013;30(2):225–36.
18. Reiley MA. INBONE total ankle replacement. Foot Ankle Spec 2008;1(5):305–8.
19. Adams SB Jr, Demetracopoulos CA, Queen RM, et al. Early to mid-term results of fixed-bearing total ankle arthroplasty with a modular intramedullary tibial component. J Bone Joint Surg Am 2014;96(23):1983–9.
20. Rush SM, Todd N. Salto Talaris fixed-bearing total ankle replacement system. Clin Podiatr Med Surg 2013;30(1):69–80.
21. Bonnin M, Gaudot F, Laurent JR, et al. The Salto total ankle arthroplasty: survivorship and analysis of failures at 7 to 11 years. Clin Orthop Relat Res 2011;469(1):225–36.
22. Bonnin M, Judet T, Colombier JA, et al. Midterm results of the Salto Total Ankle Prosthesis. Clin Orthop Relat Res 2004;(424):6–18.

Sports Medicine and Arthroscopic Treatment of the Foot and Ankle
What Is New and Current in Singapore

Sean Wei Loong HO, MBBS, MRCS (Edin)*,
Gowreeson Thevendran, MBChB (Bristol), MFSEM (UK), FRCS Ed (Tr&Orth)

KEYWORDS

• Foot and ankle • Sports • Arthroscopy • Treatment • Singapore

KEY POINTS

- Foot and ankle abnormalities are common in Singapore because of the compulsory conscription, the slipper-wearing culture, and the promotion of healthy living through exercise.
- The rapidly aging population, lack of elite sportsmen, and social and cultural norms pose unique challenges to foot and ankle surgery.
- Orthopedic surgery in Singapore has progressed because of the good infrastructure and modern practices executed by fellowship-trained surgeons.
- Evolving local practices are polarized by practice trends emulated from North America and Europe.
- The small community of foot and ankle surgeons currently practicing in Singapore allows for easier communication, corroborative educational events, and research initiatives among surgeons.

INTRODUCTION

Singapore is an independent city-state in South-east Asia. Since its independence in 1965, Singapore has developed rapidly into a modern metropolis with a population of 5.5 million people.[1] Along with Singapore's rapid development, standards in living, education, and in particular, health care have reached admirable heights. The Singapore Healthcare Model has evolved from a British-influenced system into its current state as a modern, cost-effective, and unique model. Orthopedic surgery in Singapore itself started from humble beginnings and has since progressed into a first-world service

The authors have nothing to disclose.
Department of Orthopaedic Surgery, 11 Jalan Tan Tock Seng, Tan Tock Seng Hospital, Singapore 308433, Singapore
* Corresponding author.
E-mail address: sean.ho@mohh.com.sg

Foot Ankle Clin N Am 21 (2016) 283–295
http://dx.doi.org/10.1016/j.fcl.2016.01.005
1083-7515/16/$ – see front matter © 2016 Elsevier Inc. All rights reserved.

characterized by good infrastructure and modern practices executed by surgeons incarnated from structured training programs and fellowship training from internationally acclaimed centers.

This article aims to describe the health care system and unique population challenges in Singapore and their effects on the current foot and ankle practices as well as the influences for new developments in this subspecialty.

THE SINGAPORE HEALTHCARE MODEL

The Singapore Healthcare Model consists of both a public and a private health care arm. Approximately 4% of the gross domestic product is spent on the public health care sector with the aim to provide affordable and competent health care services.[2] This model is well lauded internationally, with Singapore ranked as the world's 6th best health care system by the World Health Organization in the year 2000.[3]

The public health care system is designed to be a universal system centered around a "3M" principle: Medisave, Medishield, and Medifund. Medisave is a compulsory medical savings account contributed monthly by both the worker and their employer. This enforced savings allows for a financial safety net in the event of unforeseen medical fees. Medishield is a government-run, low-cost health insurance plan that uses the concept of risk pooling. This scheme allows Singaporeans to mitigate financial strains for large hospital bills and costly outpatient services. Finally, Medifund is a government endowment fund that can help needy patients should they require financial assistance for medical bills.

The basis of the 3M model is that of shared responsibility, copayment, and affordable health care. The copayment concept allows for a degree of cost containment because ordinary citizens often choose the most cost-efficient medical care. Translated to orthopedic surgery, this results in patients being mindful of excessive procedural as well as implant costs. Cost-effectiveness is thus an important factor in deciding the type of surgical intervention.

Health Care Facilities and Manpower

A total of 10,756 hospital beds are available in 25 public hospitals and specialty centers in Singapore.[4] Of those 25 locations, there are 6 acute general hospitals, each with its own orthopedic surgery department. The public hospital pricing serves as a benchmark for the 10 private hospitals. In terms of specialist manpower, there are 184 registered orthopedic specialists in Singapore as of 2013, with 112 (61%) in public practice.[5] As the population continues to grow and age, there is a need to increase the number of orthopedic specialists. In 2010, Singapore adopted the Accreditation Council for Graduate Medical Education (ACGME) residency system. There is now an increased number of orthopedic surgery trainees with up to 25 new orthopedic surgeons accredited yearly.

The first medical school in Singapore was founded in 1905.[6] The academic Department of Orthopaedic Surgery was founded in 1952, as a result of increased global interest in orthopedic surgery as a distinct specialty. Orthopedic sub-specialty services began in the late 1970s. Postgraduate surgical training in Singapore has historically been based on the British system, with surgical education following a British style of basic and advanced surgical specialty training. Singapore is a Royal College of Surgeons of Edinburgh–accredited orthopedic training center. Singapore-trained orthopedic surgeons can thus sit for a joint exit orthopedic examination with the Royal College of Surgeons of Edinburgh, and successful candidates can obtain an

FRCS(Edin) (fellow of the Royal College of Surgeons of Edinburgh) in Orthopaedic Surgery. This system has now given way to the new ACGME residency program.

Foot and Ankle Subspecialty

Foot and ankle surgery is a relatively young and growing orthopedic sub-speciality in Singapore. Recognizing the need for local surgeons to improve their experience and standards, the Singapore government introduced the Health Manpower Development Programme (HMDP) in the late 1980s. This HMDP fellowship was designed to allow for local surgeons to pursue fellowships at centers of excellence overseas and led to several foot and ankle surgeons completing their fellowship training in Canada or Europe. As such, there is a geographic affiliation in clinical decision-making and treatment of choice. As of 2014, there were 7 fellowship-trained foot and ankle surgeons practicing in the public sector. This small number of fellowship-trained surgeons allows for a more cohesive community with regular and convenient discussions regarding foot and ankle conditions and updates to treatment options.

PATIENT DEMOGRAPHICS

Singapore has a confluence of both Western and Asian influences. Western-styled development and practice are mired with Asian cultural beliefs. This unique mix has influenced the patients' knowledge, attitudes, and beliefs toward surgery. In addition, the tropical climate and unique social factors, such as compulsory conscription and a diminished elite sportsmen presence, affect the prevalence of foot and ankle surgery.

Compulsory Conscription

Compulsory conscription in Singapore was initiated in 1967 as a way to build a defensive force rapidly.[7] Singapore now conscripts all 18-year-old able-bodied men for 2 years. A significant percentage of new conscripts are not physically active individuals before enlistment and may not be able to adapt to the physical demands of military training. Heavy loads, prolonged boot wear, increased physical activity, and obesity have lead to an increased prevalence of foot and ankle injuries. This finding is consistent with data from the United States that showed that up to 16% of active soldiers were seen once a year for foot and ankle injuries.[8] Locally, conscripts are often open to the idea of surgery if required. First, the treatment of many foot and ankle abnormalities requires supportive footwear and physiotherapy. Although primary and even specialized medical care is readily available to conscripts, the difficulty in implementing regular physiotherapy, supportive shoe wear, and activity modification during the military training phase may blunt the effectiveness of nonsurgical treatment. Second, medical expenses during conscription are borne by the government. As such, conscripts requiring surgery are more likely to be agreeable.

Lack of Elite Sporting Culture

National campaigns detailing the benefits of sports were implemented during the early decades of independence. Sports were encouraged as a tool for improving health and fitness as well as to improve national cohesion. Over the last few decades, the focus has shifted from health benefits of sports to that of nurturing an elite sporting environment. In line with this emphasis, the first Minister of Sports was appointed in 2000. In addition, the Singapore Sports School was opened in 2004, meant as a specialized school dedicated to young sports persons.

Despite these efforts, there remain many barriers for the elite sportsman in Singapore. The lack of international success, absence of a thriving sporting culture, and poor remuneration are some reasons leading to a conspicuously low number of elite sportsmen.[9] As such, although there are elective foot and ankle sports surgeries performed for the local elite sportsman population, the rates are low as compared with the rest of the world. In addition, many local sportsmen may choose to give up or change sports after suffering foot and ankle injuries, rather than proceeding for therapeutic surgery. There are thus limited local data on the effectiveness of procedures performed in the elite sportsman population in Singapore.

Increase in Aging Population

The percentage of the world population aged 60 years and over is increasing.[10] Much like the global trend, there is an increase in the local aging population, giving rise to a "silver tsunami." Promotion of an active lifestyle coupled with increasing affluence has led to a focus on a health-conscious lifestyle with an emphasis on regular physical exercise, predisposing the elderly to foot and ankle injuries. In addition, the presence of comorbidities such as osteoporosis may also contribute to injury rates. In the geriatric population, factors such as preinjury ambulatory status and presence of comorbidities will influence the treatment options. Although the favored treatment is often nonsurgical, the growing demands of active elderly in the population suggest that the rates of surgery in these patients may increase in tandem.

Social and Cultural Norms

The social and cultural norms in Singapore play a large role in surgical treatments for foot and ankle abnormality. Local patients are strongly influenced by Asian cultural beliefs. These beliefs often lead to a low uptake in elective surgery as Singaporeans may choose to exhaust all conservative treatments before considering surgical treatment. Many patients attempt lifestyle modification rather than surgical intervention. In addition, the decision for surgery is often made in conjunction with the family. The older generation may be less enthusiastic for surgery as a result of poor prior experiences during the developing years. The older generation may also promote the use of readily available alternative therapies such as traditional ethnic medications and acupuncture. These factors affect the prevalence of surgical treatment for foot and ankle abnormalities.

CURRENT TREATMENTS

The treatment of choice for various foot and ankle abnormalities is partly influenced by surgeon preference. In the local context, most surgeons are polarized by practices adapted from their fellowship training experience. The authors surveyed 9 fellowship-trained foot and ankle surgeons (with a response rate of 6 of the 7 public sector surgeons and 2 private surgeons). They discussed details of their fellowship training, preferred surgical treatment for 4 common clinical conditions, and the rationale for their practice.

All of the surgeons surveyed underwent fellowship training in either Europe or Canada, with 66.6% of the surgeons completing a European fellowship. Among those who trained in Europe, Geneva was the most popular location. The average duration of the fellowships was 12.4 months (10–15 months). The authors noticed that no surgeons chose to do a fellowship in the United States. This finding may be influenced by 2 factors. First, most Singaporean surgeons may not choose a fellowship in the United States because of the need to obtain the USMLE (US Medical Licensing Examination) certification. Second, because of the small community, it is likely that budding foot and ankle surgeons would proceed to centers that have had positive feedback from previous local fellows. These factors may account for the current popularity of the European and Canadian training centers.

Osteochondral Lesions of the Talus

Osteochondral lesions of the talus (OLT) often occur after an episode of trauma. Patients may present with simple ankle sprains, only to return weeks later with persistent ankle swelling and pain. Khor and Tan[11] investigated 64 patients who presented with ankle sprains and found that 14% had concomitant OLTs identified on MRI. This local finding mirrors that of Roemer and colleagues,[12] who found that 7.7% of ankle sprains had concomitant OLTs. Although it is acknowledged that ankle sprains are common, the higher rate of ligamentous laxity[13] in the population may also predispose to an increased risk of musculoskeletal injuries.[14] In addition, Singaporeans often don slippers instead of supportive shoe wear due to the humid tropical weather. This habit may, in part, account for the repeated ankle sprains.

In a local study conducted by Lee,[15] up to 56% of the patients who presented to the emergency department with an acute moderate (unable to take 3 steps) ankle sprain had problems with sports 6 weeks after injury. This observation is important because of the background of compulsory conscription. Conscripts who suffer an ankle sprain may be in the midst of completing their basic/advanced military training courses. Although medical practitioners can advise them to reduce physical activity for 6 weeks, conscripts may be unwilling to do so because a prolonged absence can result in them having to repeat their training course. These conscripts may return to military training earlier than advised and predispose themselves to a repetitive injury and possible permanent instability. Multiple ankle sprains may predispose these patients to OLTs.

There are numerous treatment options for OLT injuries, with the general principle being reconstitution of the articular surface. Surgical options are dependent on several factors: namely, the degree of osseous or cartilaginous involvement, chronicity, size, and location of injury. Whenever possible, acute fixation of an osteochondral defect is ideal. If fixation cannot be achieved for the fragment, the loose fragment should be excised to prevent intra-articular pain and damage. The optimal management of lesions not amenable to direct fixation is controversial. Bone marrow stimulation results in the growth of a fibrocartilaginous plug over the lesion and has been shown to be an effective treatment. Zengerink and colleagues[16] performed a systematic review of the literature and included 52 studies in 1362 patients, showing a success rate of 85% for bone marrow stimulation in lesions up to 150 mm^2. In lesions larger than 150 mm^2, the current literature suggests there may be a less superior outcome with bone marrow stimulation alone.[16] In such lesions, other techniques may be more suitable and include autologous chondrocyte implantation, matrix-assisted autologous chondrocyte implantation, and mosaicplasty or autologous matrix-induced chondrogenesis (AMIC). Some of these techniques have been further supplemented with the use of mesenchymal stem cell usage, and this may limit its use in certain local hospitals, due to a lack of laboratory support. There is currently no compelling evidence to suggest superiority of any of the above methods.

In the authors' survey, 88.9% of the surgeons would proceed with microfracture for lesions less than 150 mm^2. For lesions larger than 150 mm^2, 55.6% of the surgeons chose to perform AMIC, with the rest performing microfracture. These results are reflective of the high reported success rate of microfracture in lesions of varying sizes. Surgeons had, however, a lower threshold to perform AMIC once the lesion size exceeded 150 mm^2.

Syndesmotic Injuries

Syndesmotic ligament injuries often occur in association with ankle trauma. Between 47% and 66% of all Weber B and C ankle fractures result in syndesmotic injuries.[17,18] Complete disruption of the syndesmosis can result in up to 40% loss of the contact surface area, potentially predisposing to early osteoarthritis.[19] There are, however, several controversies pertaining to the diagnostic and management aspects of syndesmotic injuries.

The diagnosis of a syndesmotic injury can be challenging. With complete disruption of the syndesmosis, plain radiographs may show a diastasis between the tibia and fibula with an increased medial clear space. Conversely, radiographs may be equivocal in cases of a partial syndesmotic injury. Among the local faculty, only 44.4% of surgeons recommended the use of manual stress radiographs to assist in the diagnosis of an acute syndesmotic injury, reflecting the lack of sensitivity and specificity with such maneuvers. Almost all surgeons (88.9%) performed a Cotton test intraoperatively to assess for syndesmotic injuries, citing the ease of performing this test. Most (55.6%) of the surgeons proposed direct visualization or ankle arthroscopy as a diagnostic tool for syndesmotic evaluation. None of the surgeons opted for cleaning and draping the contralateral leg for comparison, citing inconvenience as the major limiting factor.

Type and method of fixation of syndesmotic injuries remain controversial. Although there is largely an agreement that syndesmotic injuries should be treated, there appears to be no consensus if static or dynamic fixation methods should be used. Even among proponents of syndesmotic screw fixation, there is considerable variation in the size of the screw, number of screws, or the number of cortices it traverses. Advocates of the suture-button fixation technique claim their fixation is more physiologic and has the considerable advantage of not necessitating removal of fixation device. Among the local faculty, 66.6% of the surgeons preferred screw fixation to suture-button fixation. Surgeons who chose screw fixation cited reliability, cost, and quicker surgery as the main reasons for their choice. Surgeons who chose tightrope fixation substantiated their choice citing the advantage of not requiring a second operative procedure.

Os Naviculare Syndrome

The accessory navicular bone can be formed from an unfused accessory ossification center, often lying medial to the posteromedial aspect of the navicular bone. The incidence of an accessory navicular bone is reported to be from 4% to 21%.[20] Three types of accessory navicular are described based on radiological morphology. Type I is a concentric ossicle that has no contact with the proper navicular bone. Type II, which is the most common type, is separated by a fibrocartilaginous synchondrosis. Type III is an accessory navicular bone that is fused with the proper navicular bone.

The presence of an accessory navicular can lead to complaints of medial-sided foot pain. In addition, there is a possible contribution of an accessory navicular to worsening of a pes planus deformity. Patients may complain of pain over the navicular bone during activities that involve donning of stiff footwear. In the authors' population, this is especially pertinent when new recruits are exposed to increased levels of physical activity in army boots. Typically, this accentuates medial-sided pain and may lead to an incidental finding of an accessory navicular bone.

Symptomatic accessory navicular bones can often be treated conservatively. Activity modification, supportive footwear with medial insoles, and pharmacologic treatment with anti-inflammatories can help resolve the acute exacerbations.

Although these conservative treatments are effective, there are some barriers to compliance in the local setting. Because of the hot and humid weather in Singapore, there is a strong slipper-wearing culture. Patients often reject supportive shoes with medial insoles as a form of treatment because of the perceived inconvenience. In addition, activity modification during national military service may also prove to be challenging.

In cases of pain recalcitrant to conservative measures, surgery is a suitable alternative. Simple excision has been shown to produce satisfactory results, as has a modified Kidner procedure, which involves a reattachment of the posterior tibialis tendon.[21,22] Arthrodesis of the accessory navicular bone has also been attempted. This procedure involves removing the synchondrosis and fusing the accessory to the navicular bone proper with a compression screw. Results of this procedure have also been shown to be satisfactory.[23]

Among the local faculty, most of the surgeons (88.9%) chose a combination of analgesia, orthotics, and physiotherapy as their first-line choice of conservative treatment. The modified Kidner procedure was the most popular surgical choice (88.9%), with a minority of the surgeons (33.3%) considering either simple excision or fixation.

Lateral Ligament Instability

Ankle sprains are one of the more common injuries to the ankle. Ligamentous injury can occur after a sprained ankle, and in particular, the lateral ligamentous structures are the most commonly injured. The lateral ligaments include the anterior talo-fibular ligament (ATFL), calcaneo-fibular ligament, and the posterior talo-fibular ligament. The ATFL is the most commonly injured structure in ankle sprains.[24]

Acute management of ankle sprains consists of rest, cryotherapy, and elevation. Most patients will recover with appropriate rest and rehabilitation. However, 10% to 20% may develop persistent instability after repeated inversion injuries.[25,26] Repeated injuries to ligaments may also result in scar tissue formation and attenuated or torn ligaments. A torn and scarred ATFL can give rise to focal impingement pain, instability, and the potential for recurrent ankle sprains resulting in damage to the ankle joint cartilage.

There are 3 main surgical solutions for ankle instability, and these include anatomic repair, nonanatomical repair, and augmented anatomic reconstructions. The gold standard procedure for anatomic repair is the Brostrom-Gould operation. The original technique, first described by Brostrom,[27] involved taking the torn ligament ends and repairing them in a pants-over-vest fashion. In an attempt to achieve a more robust repair, Gould modified this procedure to include the plication of the extensor retinaculum to provide additional support to the repaired ankle ligaments. Results have been shown to be satisfactory.[28]

Nonanatomical repairs do not seek to re-create the original lateral ligament complex. Conversely, using other structures, this approach aims to reproduce a lateral constraint and improve stability. An example of a nonanatomical repair is the Chrisman-Snook procedure. This procedure involves using half of the peroneous brevis tendon. The tendon is harvested proximally and routed through a horizontal drill hole in the lateral malleolus. It is then passed below the peroneal tendons and into another osseous tunnel made in the calcaneum. Finally, the tendon is tensioned and stitched back onto itself. Although this procedure has been shown to be effective, complications such as overtightening of the lateral ankle have been reported.[29] Cheng and Tho[30] reported the outcomes of the Chrisman-Snook procedure in the local population and found that 14 of 15 ankles had excellent or good outcomes, similar to Snook's long-term outcomes. In addition, the investigators stated that the higher incidence of ligamentous laxity in the local population[13] may prove beneficial because it mitigates the complication of overtightness.

Augmented anatomic reconstructions focus on anatomic reconstruction of the torn or attenuated ligament; this is then combined with an autograft or allograft tissue. This method of treatment combines the benefits of an anatomic reconstruction and the additional stability that a graft confers. Yong and colleagues[31] reported the outcome of combining an anatomic reconstruction with peroneous brevis tendon augmentation in the local population. In their series of 15 patients, the mean postoperative American Orthopaedic Foot and Ankle Society (AOFAS) ankle and hindfoot score at 6 months was 91.5; 66% of their patients reported no limitation in daily and recreational activities after the operative procedure. The proposed advantage of this procedure was an early return to weight-bearing with orthotics within a week of surgery. In addition, the investigators recommended a smaller 5.5-mm interference screw be used for the augmentation procedure given the smaller fibula in the Asian population.

Among local surgeons, 77.8% chose a Bostrom-Gould repair as their surgical treatment of choice. Six of the 7 surgeons (85.6%) preferred to perform the Bostrom-Gould repair as an open procedure. This choice may be reflective of the current literature, with no compelling evidence to suggest that the arthroscopic Bostrom-Gould repair is superior to an open repair.

NEW MODALITIES OF TREATMENT IN SINGAPORE
Radiofrequency Coblation in Plantar Fasciitis

Plantar fasciitis is a degenerative condition and a common cause of heel pain. The prevalence is estimated at 10% of the general population, and this may be even higher in the athletic population.[32] The disease process is similar to tendinosis and demonstrates a lack of inflammatory cells, disorganized vascular hyperplasia, as well as an increase in disorganized collagen fibers.[33,34] Patients often complain of a sharp pain over the medial heel, typically worse after the first few steps of walking in the morning or after a long period of recumbency. Established risk factors include obesity, inadequate padding within footwear, and occupational hazards that necessitate prolonged standing (such as military personnel, construction workers, and athletes).[35]

Plantar fasciitis is known to be a self-limiting condition. Modification of aggravating risk factors can often promote recovery. However, it has been noted that these symptoms can be severely disabling, and patients are likely to demand some form of curative treatment.[36] Conservative treatment options for plantar fasciitis are well established. Plantar fascia stretching exercises have been shown to reduce symptoms.[37] Furthermore, patient education on appropriate footwear is important. In order to reduce the strain on the plantar fascia, patients should be advised to use arch supports as well as heel cups. Lee and colleagues[38] performed a meta-analysis examining the effects of orthoses on pain reduction in patients with plantar fasciitis and showed that the use of foot orthoses in patients with plantar fasciitis was associated with a reduction in pain and a functional improvement.

For patients who have persistent pain after activity modification and patient-directed therapy, the use of injections may be considered. There are several treatment modalities that include platelet-rich plasma (PRP) and corticosteroid injections. The use of autologous blood and PRP injections seeks to introduce cytokines and growth factors around the damaged tendon to generate recovery. PRP aims to deliver a greater concentration of such bioactive blood components. Monto[39] conducted a prospective randomized trial, subjecting patients to either PRP or corticosteroid injections. They showed that the PRP group had a greater increase in AOFAS scores, and these scores were maintained for longer than that of the corticosteroid group. The investigator concluded that PRP was more effective and durable than cortisone injection for the treatment of recalcitrant plantar fasciitis. Other alternative treatments to surgery include the use of low-energy extracorporeal shock-wave therapy that has also been shown to be an effective therapy.[40]

In Singapore, there has been increased interest in the use of radiofrequency microtenotomy in the treatment of plantar fasciitis. Coblation of the tendon using a radiofrequency probe can increase levels of fibroblastic growth factor and vascular endothelial growth factor, resulting in increased local angiogenesis.[41] This procedure is attractive to patients because the surgical incision required is smaller than that required for a plantar fasciotomy. Furthermore, it reduces the risk of complications associated with release of plantar fascia, namely collapse of the medial arch. Sean and colleagues[42] studied 14 local patients treated with radiofrequency coblation of the plantar fascia. They reported 12 of the 14 patients with good to excellent satisfaction at 6 months. This finding was consistent with findings from a local prospective trial conducted by Tay and colleagues.[32] They showed that patients treated with radiofrequency coblation had good expectation and satisfaction scores, with clinical results improving with time up to 1-year postoperatively. The same study concluded that the open method of coblation resulted in significantly greater improvements in pain visual analog scores (VAS) at the 1-year postoperative period when compared with the percutaneous method.

Endoscopic Gastrocnemius Recession

Increased forefoot pressures during the gait cycle have been attributed to gastrocnemius contractures.[43] The Silfverskiöld test is a clinical test for gastrocnemius tightness. Ankle dorsiflexion of less than 10° of with knee extension and a subsequent increase in dorsiflexion to more than 10° with knee flexion is positive for gastrocnemius tightness.[44] Tightness of the gastrocnemius-soleus complex has been deemed a contributory factor in various abnormalities, such as adult-acquired flatfoot deformity, hallux valgus, metatarsalgia, plantar fasciitis, and Achilles tendinopathy.[45–48]

Gastrocnemius release or recession has gained traction due to its ability to alleviate forefoot pressures. Isolated gastrocnemius recessions have been shown to be an effective procedure in reducing recalcitrant foot pain.[47] In addition, gastrocnemius recession is often performed in conjunction with other reconstructive procedures for foot and ankle abnormality. First described in 1913 by Vulpius[48] and Stoffel,[49] there are many variations of this procedure that aims to release the gastrocnemius contracture. The Strayer procedure is a variant of the gastrocnemius recession procedure that has been shown to be safe and effective.[50] Increased dorsiflexion of the ankle is obtained by releasing the gastrocnemius aponeurosis while leaving the soleus complex intact. This procedure can be performed open or endoscopically. Reported complications include sural nerve injury and incomplete release of the gastrocnemius contracture.

In the authors' survey, they established that 77.8% of the local surgeons performed a gastrocnemius recession in patients with a positive Silfverskiöld test. Of these surgeons, 55.6% (5 of 7) would perform the procedure endoscopically. Endoscopic gastrocnemius recession is increasingly common and can be performed via both a double- and a single-portal approach. For the single-portal approach, the commonly used device locally is the Smart Release Endoscopic Carpal Tunnel Release system. Results for the single-portal approach appear to be promising. Thevendran and colleagues[51] conducted a prospective study on 54 patients who underwent a single-portal endoscopic gastrocnemius recession. A total of 91% of the patients reported good or very good outcomes on the Likert scale, with immediate sural nerve dysesthesia in 5.4% of patients. Although there is a paucity of literature comparing the single-portal endoscopic approach to conventional open techniques of gastrocnemius release, the available data on the single portal endoscopic approach suggest that this approach is as safe and effective as conventional open recession techniques.

Insertional Tendoachilles Tendinopathy

Enthesopathy affecting the Achilles tendon is a common cause of posterior heel pain. Often affecting active individuals, insertional Achilles tendinosis is commonly characterized by localized tenderness over the insertion of the Achilles tendon. Patients may complain of associated swelling over the region. Over time, a Haglund deformity may develop and cause further irritation to the Achilles tendon, especially when wearing tight-fitting shoes.

Nonoperative treatments include supportive footwear, heel raises, nonsteroidal anti-inflammatory drugs, as well as physical therapy. In particular, therapy regimens such as eccentric loading exercises have been shown to be efficacious in the treatment of insertional Achilles tendinosis.[52] Other treatments such as extracorporeal shock-wave therapy have also shown promising results.[53] In the local population, symptoms may be recalcitrant due to poor compliance with supportive footwear and heel raises. In those cases with recalcitrant pain, surgery may be considered.

The goals of surgery are to decompress the inflamed bursa, debride the degenerative tendon, and excise the osseous deformities that may be causing irritation. Debridement of the degenerative tendon and excision of calcaneal prominence can be achieved via both open and endoscopic means. In addition to tendon debridement, reattachment of the Achilles tendon after calcaneoplasty can also be performed, and this procedure has been shown to be effective in providing good pain relief.[54] Locally, Lin and colleagues[55] published a series of 22 patients who were treated for insertional Achilles tendinopathy with a lateral approach calcaneoplasty and reattachment of Achilles tendon. In this series, there were significant improvements in the VAS, AOFAS, and SF-36 (Short Form-36) score up to 6 months after surgery. This local study mirrors other published data[54,56] and affirms that reattachment of the Achilles tendon with calcaneoplasty is an effective treatment of insertional Achilles tendinopathy.

SUMMARY

Despite a distinct lack of elite sportsmen, foot and ankle abnormalities are relatively common in Singapore because of compulsory conscription, the slipper-wearing culture, and the promotion of healthy living through exercise. As with most developed countries worldwide, orthopedic surgical care in Singapore is delivered largely by sub-specialty practitioners. As a fraternity, the foot and ankle subspecialty is growing in Singapore, with most practicing surgeons having completed their fellowship training overseas. As such, evolving local practices have been polarized by practice trends emulated from North America and Europe. The evolution of treatment options in Singapore has been largely propelled by evidence-based practice. Given the small community of foot and ankle surgeons currently practicing in Singapore, communication among surgeons, corroborative educational events, and research initiatives have been easier to accomplish. These practices are likely to develop tangentially in the future because Singapore continues to develop into a center of clinical excellence in the region.

REFERENCES

1. Singapore Department of Statistics. Population Trends 2014.
2. Healthcare Financing Philosophy. 2015. Available at: www.moh.gov.sg/content/moh_web/home/costs_and_financing.html. Accessed December 2014.
3. Musgrove P, Creese A, Preker A, et al. The World Health Report 2000; Health systems: improving performance. Geneva (Switzerland): World Health Organization; 2000. p. 154. ISBN 92-4-156198-X.
4. Hospital Services. 2015. Available at: www.moh.gov.sg/content/moh_web/home/our_healthcare_system/Healthcare_Services/Hospitals.html. Accessed December 2014.
5. Singapore Medical Council. (2014). 2014 Annual report of Singapore Medical Council. Available at: http://www.healthprofessionals.gov.sg/content/dam/hprof/smc/docs/annual_reports/SMC%20AR%202014-NEW%20Full-draft%2010%20-%206%20July.pdf. Accessed December 2015.
6. Wang W, Lee EH, Wong HK. One hundred years of orthopaedic education in Singapore. Ann Acad Med Singapore 2005;34(6):130C–6C.
7. Army Museum of Singapore. Available at: www.mindef.gov.sg/imindef/mindef_websites/atozlistings/army/microsites/armymuseum/stories/Personal_Stories/The_Swinging_60s.html. Accessed December 2014.
8. Wallace RF, Wahi MM, Hill OT, et al. Rates of ankle and foot injuries in active-duty U.S. Army soldiers, 2000-2006. Mil Med 2011;176(3):283–90.
9. Teo L. Comparative elite sport development: systems, structures and public policy. Oxford (UK): Elsevier; 2008. p. 84–114.
10. United Nations, Department of Economic and Social Affairs, Population Division (2013). United Nations (New York): World Population Ageing; 2013.
11. Khor YP, Tan KJ. The anatomic pattern of injuries in acute inversion ankle sprains: a magnetic resonance imaging study. Orthop J Sports Med 2013;1(7). 2325967113517078.
12. Roemer FW, Jomaah N, Niu J, et al. Ligamentous injuries and the risk of associated tissue damage in acute ankle sprains in athletes: a cross-sectional MRI study. Am J Sports Med 2014;42(7):1549–57.
13. Seow CC, Chow PK, Khong KS. A study of joint mobility in a normal population. Ann Acad Med Singapore 1999;28(2):231–6.
14. Razak HR, Ali NB, Howe TS. Generalized ligamentous laxity may be a predisposing factor for musculoskeletal injuries. J Sci Med Sport 2014;17:474–8.
15. Lee WY. Audit on treatment and recovery of ankle sprain. Hong Kong J Emerg Med 2002;9(2):72–7.
16. Zengerink M, Struijs PA, Tol JL, et al. Treatment of osteochondral lesions of the talus: a systematic review. Knee Surg Sports Traumatol Arthrosc 2010;18(2):238–46.
17. Loren GJ, Ferkel RD. Arthroscopic assessment of occult intra-articular injury in acute ankle fractures. Arthroscopy 2002;18(4):412–21.
18. Th Lui, Ip K, Chow HT. Comparison of radiologic and arthroscopic diagnoses of distal tibiofibular syndesmosis disruption in acute ankle fracture. Arthroscopy 2005;21(11):1370.
19. Ramsey PL, Hamilton W. Changes in tibiotalar area of contact caused by lateral talar shift. J Bone Joint Surg Am 1976;58:356–7.
20. Lee KT, Kim KC, Park YU, et al. Midterm outcome of modified Kidner procedure. Foot Ankle Int 2012;33(2):122–7.

21. Jasiewicz B, Potaczek T, Kacki W, et al. Results of simple excision technique in the surgical treatment of symptomatic accessory navicular bones. Foot Ankle Surg 2008;14(2):57–61.
22. Micheli LJ, Nielson JH, Ascani C, et al. Treatment of painful accessory navicular: a modification to simple excision. Foot Ankle Spec 2008;1(4):214–7.
23. Scott AT, Sabesan VJ, Saluta JR, et al. Fusion versus excision of the symptomatic type II accessory navicular: a prospective study. Foot Ankle Int 2009;30(1):10–5.
24. Malliaropoulos N, Ntessalen M, Papacostas E, et al. Reinjury after acute lateral ankle sprains in elite track and field athletes. Am J Sports Med 2009;37:1755–61.
25. Harrington KD. Degenerative arthritis of the ankle secondary to long-standing lateral ligament instability. J Bone Joint Surg Am 1979;61:354–61.
26. Sammarco GJ, DiRaimondo CV. Surgical treatment of lateral ankle instability syndrome. Am J Sports Med 1988;16:501–11.
27. Brostrom L. Sprained ankles. VI. Surgical treatment of 'chronic' ligament ruptures. Acta Chir Scand 1966;132:551–65.
28. Hamilton WG, Thompson FM, Snow SW. The modified Brostrom procedure for lateral ankle instability. Foot Ankle 1993;14:1–7.
29. Dalal RB, Sian P, Mahajan R. The modified Chrisman Snook procedure for chronic lateral instability of the ankle—long-term results. J Bone Joint Surg Br 2008;90B:498.
30. Cheng M, Tho KS. Chrisman-Snook ankle ligament reconstruction outcomes—a local experience. Singapore Med J 2002;43(12):605–9.
31. Yong R, Lai KW, Ooi LH. Ankle lateral ligament reconstruction for chronic instability. J Orthop Surg (Hong Kong) 2015;23(1):62–5.
32. Tay KS, Ng YC, Singh IR, et al. Open technique is more effective than percutaneous technique for TOPAZ radiofrequency coblation for plantar fasciitis. Foot Ankle Surg 2012;18(4):287–92.
33. Almekinders LC. Tendinitis and other chronic tendinopathies. J Am Acad Orthop Surg 1998;6:157–64.
34. Tasto JP, Cummings J, Medlock V, et al. Microtenotomy using a radiofrequency probe to treat lateral epicondylitis. Arthroscopy 2005;21(7):851–60.
35. Beeson P. Plantar fasciopathy: revisiting the risk factors. Foot Ankle Surg 2014;20(3):160–5.
36. League AC. Current concepts review—plantar fasciitis. Foot Ankle Int 2008;29:358–66.
37. Hyland MR, Webber-Gaffney A, Cohen L, et al. Randomized controlled trial of calcaneal taping, sham taping, and plantar fascia stretching for the short-term management of plantar heel pain. J Orthop Sports Phys Ther 2006;36(6):364–71.
38. Lee SY, McKeon P, Hertel J. Does the use of orthoses improve self-reported pain and function measures in patients with plantar fasciitis? A meta-analysis. Phys Ther Sport 2009;10(1):12–8.
39. Monto RR. Platelet-rich plasma efficacy versus corticosteroid injection treatment for chronic severe plantar fasciitis. Foot Ankle Int 2014;35(4):313–8.
40. Rompe JD, Kullmer K, Riehle HM, et al. Effectiveness of low-energy extracorporeal shock waves for chronic plantar fasciitis. Foot Ankle Surg 1996;2:215–21.
41. Dietz U, Horstick G, Manke T, et al. Myocardial angiogenesis resulting in functional communications with the left cavity induced by intramyocardial high-frequency ablation: histomorphology of immediate and long-term effects in pigs. Cardiology 2003;99:32–8.
42. Sean NY, Singh I, Wai CK. Radiofrequency microtenotomy for the treatment of plantar fasciitis shows good early results. Foot Ankle Surg 2010;16(4):174–7.

43. Macklin K, Healy A, Chockalingam N. The effect of calf muscle stretching exercises on ankle joint dorsiflexion and dynamic foot pressures, force and related temporal parameters. Foot (Edinb) 2012;22(1):10–7.
44. Singh D. Nils Silfverskiold (1999-1957) and gastrocnemius contracture. Foot Ankle Surg 2013;19(2):135–8.
45. Aronow MS, Diaz-Doran V, Sullivan RJ, et al. The effect of triceps surae contracture force on plantar foot pressure distribution. Foot Ankle Int 2006;27(1):43–52.
46. Downey MS, Banks AS. Gastrocnemius recession in the treatment of nonspastic ankle equinus. A retrospective study. J Am Podiatr Med Assoc 1989;79(4): 159–74.
47. Maskill JD, Bohay DR, Anderson JG. Gastrocnemius recession to treat isolated foot pain. Foot Ankle Int 2010;31(1):19–23.
48. Takahashi S, Shrestha A. The Vulpius procedure for correction of equinus deformity in patients with hemiplegia. J Bone Joint Surg Br 2002;84(7):978–80.
49. Stoffel A. The treatment of spastic contractures. J Bone Joint Surg 1913;210(4): 611–44.
50. Pinney SJ, Hansen ST Jr, Sangeorzan BJ. The effect of ankle dorsiflexion on gastrocnemius recession. Foot Ankle Int 2002;23(1):26–9.
51. Thevendran G, Howe LB, Kaliyaperumal K, et al. Endoscopic gastrocnemius recession procedure using a single portal technique: a prospective study of fifty four consecutive patients. Int Orthop 2015;39(6):1099–107.
52. Kedia M, Williams M, Jain L, et al. The effects of conventional physical therapy and eccentric strengthening for insertional Achilles tendinopathy. Int J Sports Phys Ther 2014;9(4):488–97.
53. Al-Abbad H, Simon JV. The effectiveness of extracorporeal shock wave therapy on chronic Achilles tendinopathy: a systematic review. Foot Ankle Int 2013; 34(1):33–41.
54. Johnson KW, Zalavras C, Thordarson DB. Surgical management of insertional calcific achilles tendinosis with a central tendon splitting approach. Foot Ankle Int 2006;27:245–50.
55. Lin HA, Chong HA, Yeo W. Calcaneoplasty and reattachment of the Achilles tendon for insertional tendinopathy. J Orthop Surg (Hong Kong) 2014;22(1):56–9.
56. Wagner E, Gould JS, Kneidel M, et al. Technique and results of Achilles tendon detachment and reconstruction for insertional Achilles tendinosis. Foot Ankle Int 2006;27(9):677–84.

My Experience as a Foot and Ankle Trauma Surgeon in Montreal, Canada

What's Not in the Books

Stéphane Leduc, MD, FRCSC[a,b,*], Marie-Lyne Nault, MD, PhD, FRCS[a,b,c],
Dominique M. Rouleau, MD, FRCSC, MSc[a,b],
Jonah Hebert-Davies, MD, FRCSC[a,b]

KEYWORDS

- Foot trauma • Ankle trauma • Talus • Calcaneus • Tips and tricks

KEY POINTS

- Although ankle fractures are common and usually simple to treat, there are several potentially complex injuries that require special attention.
- Talar fractures are common high-energy fractures characterized by a high degree of comminution, large displacement, and significant soft tissue injury.
- Anatomic open reduction with internal fixation is the goal of calcaneal fractures, although the high-energy nature of some of these injuries makes them surgically challenging and technically complex.

INTRODUCTION: NATURE OF THE PROBLEM

One of the most challenging aspects of a foot and ankle practice is learning to address the vast number of uncommon disorders that are generally not discussed in regular textbooks and that make returning patients to previous function following foot trauma demanding. Obtaining good outcomes can be helped with meticulous preoperative evaluation, surgical planning, and optimal surgical technique. This article uses illustrative cases to provide tips to avoid the common complications and facilitate the surgical process. Four injury types are reviewed: the nonsimple ankle fracture, the talus fracture, the calcaneus fracture, and the midfoot injury.

Disclosure: Hôpital du Sacré-Cœur de Montréal has received funding from: Arthrex, Conmed, Depuy, Smith and Nephew, Stryker, Synthes, Tornier, Zimmer. S. Leduc is a consultant for Stryker.
[a] Hôpital du Sacré-Cœur de Montréal, 5400 Boulevard Gouin Ouest, Montréal, Québec H4J 1C5, Canada; [b] Department of Surgery, Université de Montréal, Québec, Canada; [c] CHU Ste-Justine, 3175 ch. De la Côte Ste-Catherine, Montréal, Québec H3T 1C5, Canada
* Corresponding author.
E-mail address: stephaneleduc@hotmail.com

THE NONSIMPLE ANKLE FRACTURE
Background

Although ankle fractures are common and usually simple to treat, there are several potentially complex injuries that require special attention. The primary goal of ankle fracture treatment is recreating normal anatomy with a centered tibiotalar joint. This article discusses several techniques to help avoid potential pitfalls.

Preoperative Assessment

1. Not all ankle fractures require surgery. However, those that do should be easily identified (**Box 1**).
2. Syndesmotic integrity cannot be evaluated solely based on fracture pattern. Although Weber type C fractures are generally associated with syndesmotic disruption, more than half of Weber type B fractures also have syndesmotic injuries.[1] Any fracture pattern with potential syndesmosis incompetency should undergo thorough intraoperative testing.
3. Preoperative computed tomography (CT) scan is useful after initial reduction, for both subtle (posterior malleolus) and complex (tibial plafond) fractures. CT helps to evaluate articular impaction and interfragmentary debris, and allows the surgeon to plan both surgical approach and fixation strategy (**Fig. 1**).
4. Soft tissue status should dictate the timing of definitive fixation. Although acute open reduction and internal fixation (ORIF) may be successful in carefully selected patients, the authors opt for fixation following normalization of soft tissues. Any grossly displaced or unstable pilon fracture should be initially treated with an external fixator to allow soft tissue swelling to resolve. Pins are placed far from the zone of injury so as not to interfere with definitive surgery. A standard delta frame is augmented with a pin in the foot (first metatarsal or cuneiforms) to control sagittal plane deformity and ensure adequate dorsiflexion.

Box 1
Surgical indication of an ankle fracture

- Open fractures
- Bimalleolar fracture and bimalleolar-equivalent fracture
- Medial malleolar displacement greater than 2 mm or lateral malleolar displacement greater than 3 mm
- Any coronal plane tibiotalar malalignment (medial clear space > superior joint space)
- Any fibular shortening
- Syndesmotic injury
- Significant posterior malleolar fracture (>25%, >2-mm step-off, or syndesmotic equivalent)
- Marginal impaction of the tibial articular surface
- Displaced intra-articular fractures of the tibial plafond
- Malalignment of the distal tibial articular surface
- Dynamic instability based on stress views

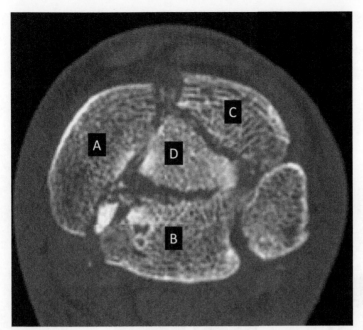

Fig. 1. Typical pilon fracture anatomy involves 4 fragments: medial malleolar (A), posterolateral/Volkmann fragment (B), anterolateral/Chaput fragment (C), and the central/die-punch fragment (D).

Tips and Tricks

Patient positioning

1. The supine position is versatile and adequate for most fractures. In general, a towel bump is placed under the ipsilateral buttock to provide neutral rotation of the ankle. However, in instances in which a posteromedial approach must also be performed, the bump is removed after lateral side fixation and the leg is positioned in a figure of 4 to allow adequate access.
2. Elevate the affected leg on a radiolucent platform. With the fluoroscopy machine positioned on the contralateral side, this facilitates obtaining good quality lateral views without manipulating the leg.

Surgical Approach

1. Multiple incisions may be necessary. With careful attention to soft tissue management and surgical timing, incisions for tibial plafond fractures may be placed less than 7 cm apart, allowing the surgeon to optimize exposures from the injury pattern. Then, the length of the incisions should be as short as possible.
2. Standard lateral and medial approaches are workhorses. These approaches allow excellent exposure of the fibula, the syndesmosis, the anterolateral part of the tibia, and the medial malleolus.
3. The approach for articular fixation should be dictated by fracture pattern. The anterior approach, between the tibialis anterior tendon and the extensor hallucis longus tendon, allows exposure of the complete anterior tibial plafond. The anterolateral approach, lateral to the anterior compartment, allows exposure of most of the anterior tibial plafond, the syndesmosis joint, and even the anterior fibula (**Fig. 2**).

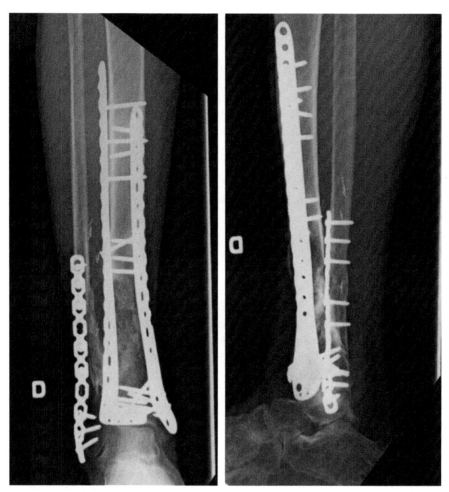

Fig. 2. Anterior fibula plating performed through an anterolateral approach of the ankle in a patient with bad soft tissue injury.

The anteromedial approach, medial to the tibialis anterior tendon, allows excellent exposure to the tibial plafond and the medial gutter.

4. Supplemental posterior approaches should be used if incomplete reduction is achieved through standard approaches. The posteromedial approach, through the posterior tibialis tendon sheath, allows exposure of the medial malleolus and most of the posterior distal tibia (**Fig. 3**). The posterolateral approach to the fibula and posterior tibia, between the peroneal tendons and the flexor hallucis longus, allows visualization of the fibula and posterior tibia.

Reduction and Fixation

1. Bicortical medial malleolar screws can be used in patients with weak bone. This method has been shown to be biomechanically stronger and lead to fewer failures.[2]
2. Atypical medial malleolus fractures deserve atypical approaches and fixation. The variant posteromedial ankle fracture must be recognized and fixed through a

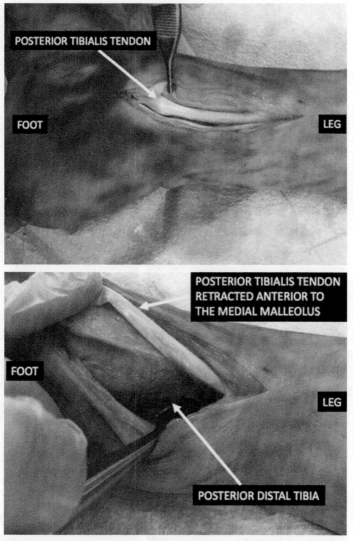

Fig. 3. Posteromedial approach through the posterior tibialis tendon sheath gives great exposure to the posterior distal tibia.

posteromedial approach (**Fig. 4**). Vertical shear medial malleolus fractures should be addressed similarly to a Schatzker 2 tibial plateau fracture with restoration of joint surface and antiglide plate (**Fig. 5**).

3. Lateral malleolus fracture requires anatomic reduction. Recreating normal length, alignment, and rotation of the fibula serves as a guide for reduction of the tibial fracture. The authors prefer posterior antiglide plating because it is biomechanically superior to lateral plating. In some severely comminuted fractures, the distal fibula can be reduced to the distal tibia with Kirschner wires (K-wires) and then fixed using a bridge plating technique (**Fig. 6**). On occasion, rafting screws can be used as well to support highly comminuted fractures (**Fig. 7**).

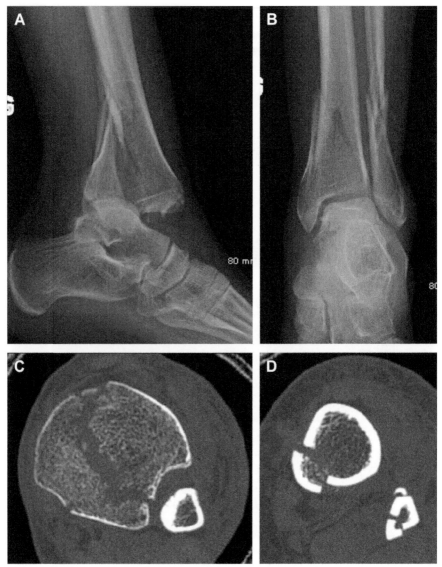

Fig. 4. Radiographs (*A*, *B*) showing an atypical posteromedial ankle fracture. Axial CT scan views near the joint (*C*) and at the apex of the fracture (*D*) confirming the fracture pattern. Radiographs (*E*, *F*) showing the ORIF through a posteromedial approach.

4. Syndesmotic reduction must be done under direct visualization. Malreduction of the syndesmotic joint is frequent.[3] The syndesmosis can be seen through the lateral fibula approach by elevating anteriorly over the ligaments (**Fig. 8**). Malreduction of the fibula fracture or incarcerated bone debris may prevent anatomic reduction of the syndesmosis and should be addressed (**Figs. 9 and 10**).

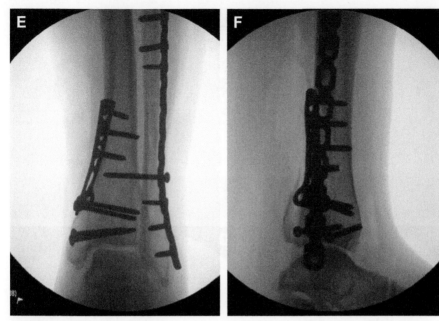

Fig. 4. (*continued*).

5. An external fixator or universal bone distractor is an excellent reduction tool. Distractors are particularly useful in tibial plafond fractures because they allow intra-articular visualization. They are also useful when treating malunions that have healed in a shortened position in order to regain appropriate length (**Fig. 11**).
6. Basic principles of periarticular fractures apply to the management of tibial plafond fractures. The goals of the procedure are anatomic reduction of the articular surface, restoration of length, bone grafting, and securing the metaphysis to the diaphysis (**Box 2, Fig. 12**).
7. Dual posterior and anterior approaches are occasionally needed. Incarcerated posterior fragments with nerve injury are a definite indication (**Fig. 13**).

Postoperative care and complications

1. Patients are immobilized in a bulky splint for 10 to 14 days. Sutures are removed when incisions are healed and gentle range of motion is begun.
2. Partial weight bearing is started at 2 weeks for malleolar fractures with progression over 6 weeks. For tibial plafond fractures, partial weight bearing is started at 6 weeks and progressed to full weight bearing at 12 weeks.
3. Patients with diabetic neuropathy should be immobilized and protected from weight bearing for twice as long as normally recommended. Wound complication and deep infection can be minimized with thorough soft tissue management. Posttraumatic arthritis is uncommon with anatomic reduction and fixation. Corrective osteotomy is recommended for optimal outcomes in cases with significant malunion and may require tricortical iliac bone graft (**Fig. 14**).[4]

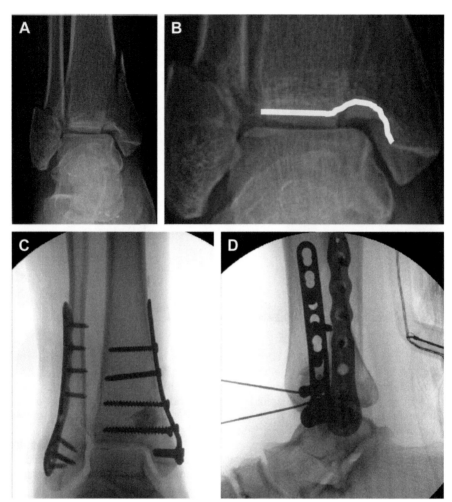

Fig. 5. AP (*A*) and zoomed AP (*B*) radiographs of a marginal medial plafond impaction (*yellow line*). Fluoroscopy (*C*, *D*) of the procedure that involved disimpaction, anatomic reduction, temporary Kirschner wires (K-wires) followed by lag screws, rafting screws, buttress plate, and grafting.

TALUS FRACTURES
Background

Talar fractures are common high-energy fractures. They can involve the body, the neck, the head, or a combination of all of these. Typical features of these fractures are a high degree of comminution, large displacement, and significant soft tissue injury. Because of the high-energy trauma necessary to cause these fractures, associated life-threatening injuries, and the soft tissue damage, definitive treatment is often delayed. Surgeons must have many different options and techniques to assist reduction in order to obtain a satisfactory result. Several of these techniques are discussed in more detail later.

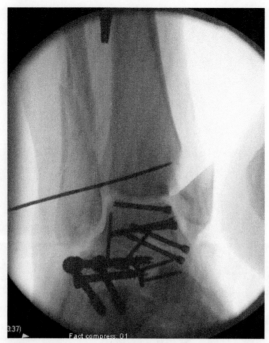

Fig. 6. K-wire temporary stabilization of the distal fibula to the tibia distal to maintain fibula length and rotation before definitive fixation.

Preoperative Assessment

Management of patients with talar fractures should be systematic to avoid complications.

1. Acute treatment should consist of closed reduction in the emergency department if possible. Any wounds are cleaned and the ankle is splinted.
2. Open fractures should undergo operative irrigation and debridement in an emergent fashion. Irreducible closed fractures should also be taken to the operating room emergently.
3. When associated injuries prevent acute definitive fixation, fractures are temporarily stabilized using external fixation and/or K-wires.
4. Preoperative imaging should include good-quality radiographs of the ankle and foot. A CT scan of the talus with coronal and sagittal reconstruction helps to evaluate fracture patterns and plan surgical approaches and fixation strategies.
5. Soft tissue swelling is allowed to dissipate before definitive surgery to avoid healing complications.

Tips and Tricks

Patient positioning

1. Always plan positioning for possible approaches. Almost all talar fractures can be operated on through anterior incisions. The patient is placed in the supine position on a radiolucent table. It often helps to place a radiolucent ramp or bumps under

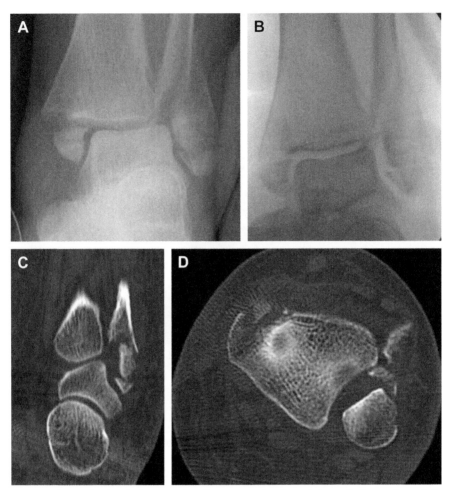

Fig. 7. Radiographs (*A–D*) showing significant comminution of the articular surface of the fibula. Radiographs (*E–G*) showing fixation with rafting screws supporting the significant articular comminution of the distal fibula.

the leg to slightly flex the knee and release tension in the gastrocnemius. If a supplementary posteromedial incision is thought to be necessary, a bump can also be placed under the contralateral hip to increase internal rotation and allow the affected side to be placed in a figure of 4.

Surgical Approach

1. Almost always uses 2 approaches. Although most fractures require exposure from dual incisions, they are especially useful for surgeons who do not routinely fix talus fractures. The anterolateral approach extends from the anterior aspect of the distal fibula to the base of the fourth metacarpal. It can be extended proximally to aid in retracting the extensor tendons. The superficial peroneal nerve must be carefully protected throughout surgery. The anteromedial approach runs from the medial

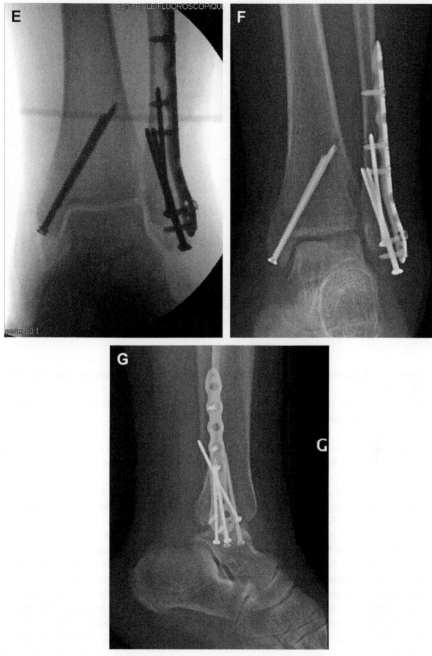

Fig. 7. (*continued*).

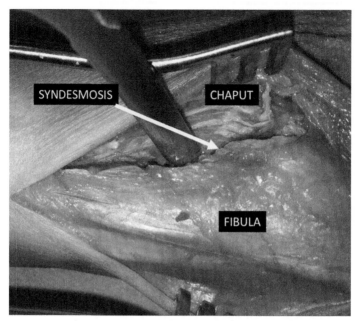

Fig. 8. Lateral approach to the ankle showing a retractor in the syndesmotic joint.

malleolus, between the tibialis posterior and tibialis anterior, to the navicular (**Fig. 15**).

2. When necessary, do not hesitate to use a medial malleolus osteotomy. Talar neck and body fractures with posterior extension can be difficult to visualize from standard approaches. In these cases, the medial malleolus osteotomy, combined with plantar flexion, allows for adequate visualization. If the deltoid ligament is torn, the vascular supply to the malleolus may be disrupted and an osteotomy is not advised. If an osteotomy is being considered, the skin incision is translated slightly posterior to allow adequate access for preparation and fixation of the osteotomy (**Fig. 16**). It is also possible to work through a fibular facture to access the lateral part of the talus (**Fig. 17**).

3. A posteromedial approach is useful for very posterior fractures. In some cases, the talus body is fractured at its most posterior border. These small fragments are difficult to fix from an anterior approach, even with a medial malleolus osteotomy. In these cases, a posterior medial approach, between the medial malleolus and the Achilles tendon, can be used. Deep dissection is performed between the flexor digitorum longus and the neurovascular bundle or between the flexor hallucis longus and the Achilles tendon. The ankle is dorsiflexed to increase visualization and fragments are fixed using mini–fragment screws or plates (**Fig. 18**).

Reduction

1. An external fixator can help reduction. In many high-energy talus fractures, soft tissues and delay from time of injury make regaining appropriate length difficult. An intraoperative external fixator helps distract the ankle and subtalar joints. A simple frame, with a medial pin in the tibia, a medial pin in the

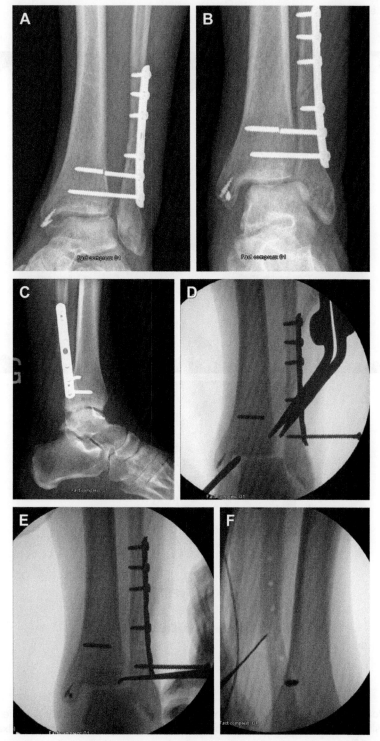

Fig. 9. Radiographs (*A–C*) showing a malreduced syndesmosis with a fibula malunion. In a chronic situation, in addition to the correction of the fibula malunion (*F*), the soft tissue interposition in the syndesmosis (*E*) and medial gutter (*D*) needs to be removed to recreate normal anatomy. Radiographs (*G–I*) showing the corrected ankle.

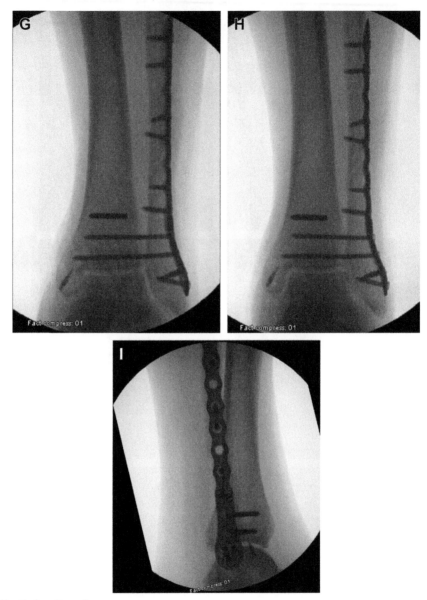

Fig. 9. (*continued*).

calcaneus, and a pin in the cuneiforms or navicular, is usually sufficient. If desired, the frame can be left on after surgery to help off-load the fixation (**Fig. 19**).
2. Avoid over-reducing the medial side. Typically, talar neck fractures have increased comminution in the posterior medial neck, which can lead to overcompression of the medial side and varus malreduction. While working through the medial

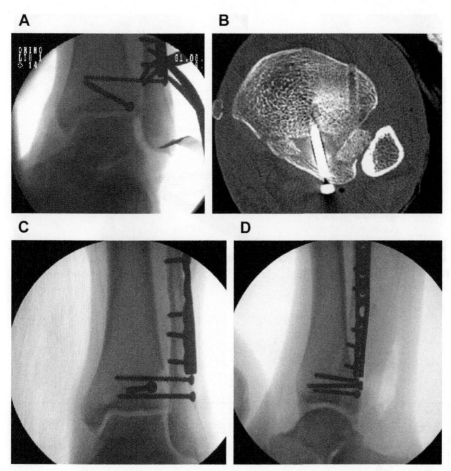

Fig. 10. Malreduced syndesmosis secondary to bone debris in the joint (*A, B*). Radiographs (*C, D*) after removal of the fragment and revision ORIF through the Bohler approach.

approach, only an approximate reduction is obtained. Then, working back and forth between the medial and lateral approaches, the definitive reduction can be achieved (**Fig. 20**). In addition, on fluoroscopic evaluation, the first metatarsal and the talar neck should be aligned on both the anteroposterior (AP) and lateral views (**Fig. 21**).
3. Disimpaction of a talar dome impaction may be performed through a cortical bone window. As for a Schatzker type 3 tibial plateau fracture, fracture disimpaction can be performed through a cortical bone window (**Fig. 22**).

Fixation

1. Plates are an excellent adjunct for fixation. In some cases, screw fixation alone is sufficient to maintain reduction of talar fractures. However, in most cases, a mini–fragment plate is necessary. Plates are usually placed on the lateral side with screws directed into the head and into the body. If more fixation is

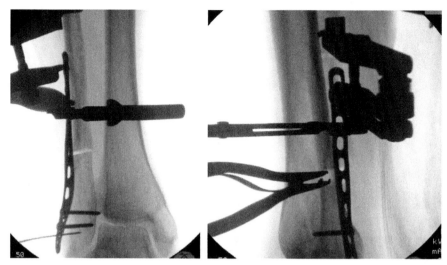

Fig. 11. Lengthening of the fibula obtained with the help of a universal distractor and a laminar spreader.

Box 2
Surgical steps for C3 pilon fracture involving a displaced posterior fragment

- Surgical exposure through an anterior approach between the anterior tibialis and extensor hallucis longus tendons (see **Fig. 12**).
- Reduce and instrument fibula to establish lateral column length.
- Reduce articular surface.
- Open the fracture like a book by reclining the anterolateral fragment laterally.
- Remove the middle fragment.
- It is important to remove interfragmentary debris with a dental pick to permit proper reduction without a gap.
- Reduce the posterior fragment by recreating its anatomy in relationship to the posterior metaphyseal tibia. It is important to reduce it adequately in the sagittal plane to prevent extension malunion. Using a K-wire as a joystick helps reduce the posterior fragment to its normal anatomy.
- Temporary stabilize with K-wire from the proximal anterior tibia to the distal posterior fragment.
- Reduce the middle fragment to the posterior distal fragment and stabilize it with K-wire.
- Reduce the medial and the anterolateral fragments and stabilize them with K-wire.
- Replace K-wire by interfragmentary screws (2.7 mm or 3.5 mm).
- Reattach articular block to metaphysis and shaft with a variable locking periarticular pilon plate.

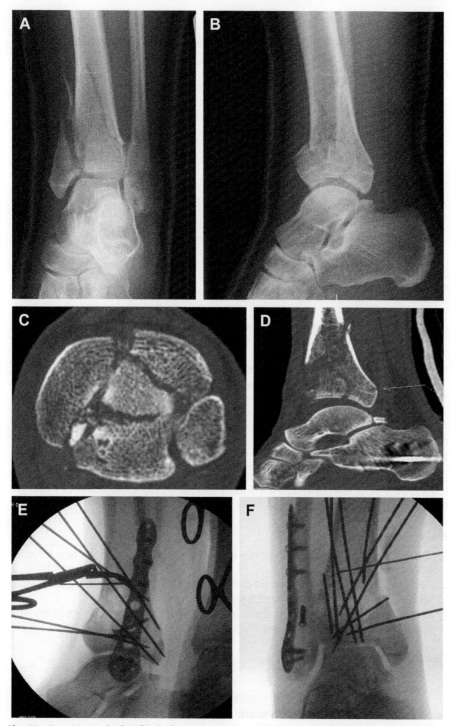

Fig. 12. Comminuted pilon fibula fractures (*A, B*). CT scan views (*C, D*) showing the displaced posterior fragment (*arrow*). Fluoroscopy (*E, F*) showing temporary stabilization of all fragments with K-wires, and the final result (*G, H*) after ORIF.

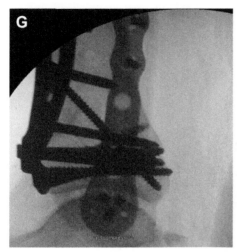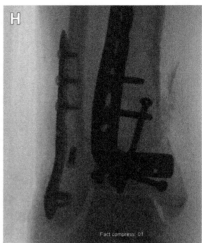

Fig. 12. (*continued*).

required, a small T plate can be used. Locking plates, although generally not required, can resist deforming forces by maintaining a length-stable construct (**Fig. 23**).
2. Not all talus fractures can be reconstructed. In rare cases of extreme comminution or infection from contaminated open fractures, sometimes the best option is a salvage procedure (**Fig. 24**).

CALCANEUS FRACTURES
Background

Calcaneus fractures are the most common tarsal fracture and are a result of axial loading trauma. Understanding the anatomy and the 5 classic fragments of this injury (**Fig. 25**) is the key to treating them.[5]

Preoperative Assessment

1. Systematic work-up and preoperative assessment should be done as described for talus fractures.
2. Because of the high-energy nature of these injuries, look for commonly associated injuries (eg, pilon fractures, spinal fractures).
3. Significantly displaced tongue-type fractures are at risk for skin necrosis and should be taken to the operating room emergently.

Tips and Tricks

Patient positioning

1. Always plan positioning for all possible approaches. Most calcaneus fractures can be operated on through a lateral extensile approach. The patient is placed in the lateral position on a radiolucent table, with the affected foot supported. However, if additional medial or posterior approaches are needed, the surgeon should ensure the patient has enough hip external rotation to allow for this.

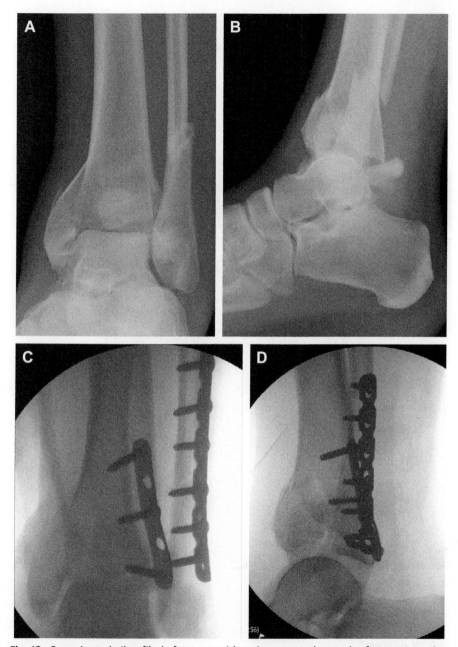

Fig. 13. Comminuted pilon fibula fractures with an incarcerated posterior fragment causing a nerve injury (*A, B*). Radiographs (*C, D*) after ORIF of the fibula and posterior part of the pilon through a posterolateral approach. Radiographs (*E, F*) showing progressive ORIF in a second stage through an anterior approach, and the final result (*G, H*).

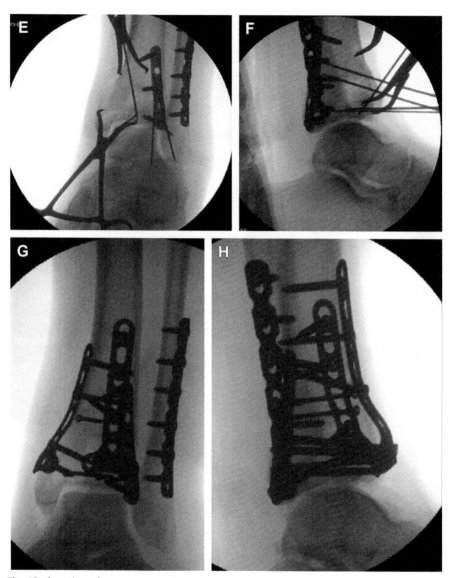

Fig. 13. (continued).

Surgical Approach

1. The extensile lateral approach is still the workhorse approach. Protecting the vascularity of the lateral flap with minimal manipulation of the skin edges is paramount to prevent necrosis. Sufficient deep exposure is crucial to complete the subtalar arthrotomy and allow proper visualization of the posterior facet reduction.

2. Sinus tarsi approach is a useful alternative to percutaneous techniques. It provides an excellent view of the subtalar joint and puts the soft

tissues at lesser risk. It should be reserved for cases that are amenable to this exposure.

Reduction

1. Do not lose focus on reduction goals. Calcaneus fractures are often very comminuted and restoring normal anatomy may be difficult. Surgeons should attempt anatomic reduction of the posterior, middle, and anterior facets; recreate calcaneal height, width, and Bohler angle; correct hind foot varus; and recreate the angle of Gissane. It is important not to focus solely on articular congruity at the expense of all these other deformities.
2. Converting a tongue-type fracture to a split depression fracture can be useful in difficult fracture dislocations.[6] Using an osteotome, the large tuberosity fragment

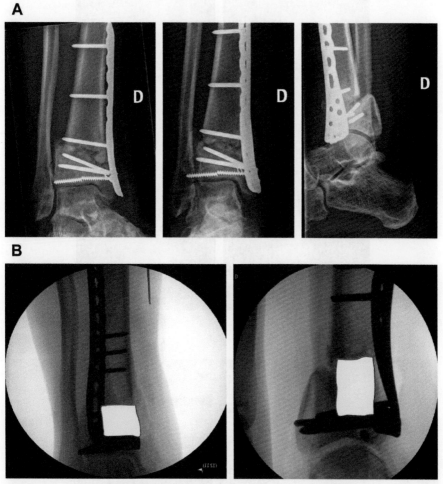

Fig. 14. Ankle views (*A*) showing a malunion nonunion of the distal metaphyseal region of the distal tibia in a 30-year-old patient. Ankle views (*B*) during the procedure with the tricortical iliac graft highlighted in yellow. Multiple views (*C*) at 4 months showing the consolidation.

C

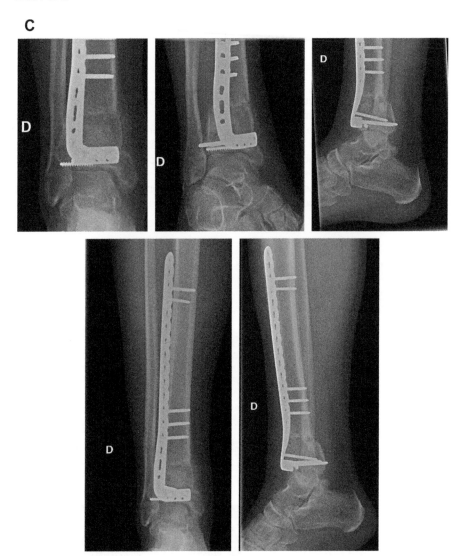

Fig. 14. (*continued*).

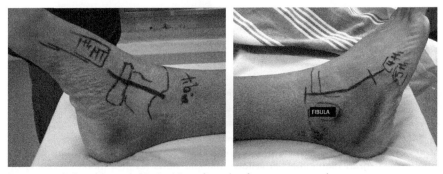

Fig. 15. Medial and lateral skin incisions for talus fracture approaches.

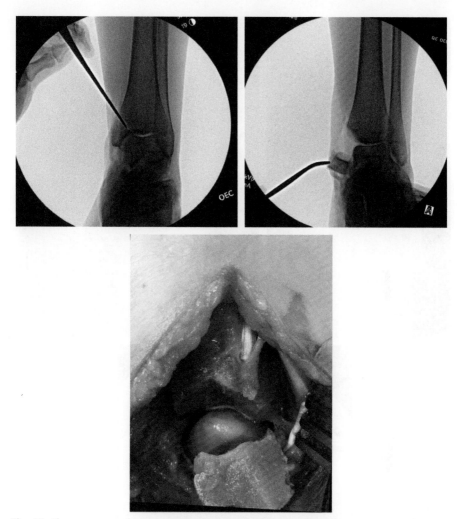

Fig. 16. Fluoroscopy and intraoperative views of medial malleolus osteotomy.

is split at the level of the posterior facet. This step simplifies exposure and reduction of the posterior facet once the tuberosity fragment is reduced posteriorly (**Fig. 26**).
3. Always have multiple reduction tools available. Schanz pins, small and large reduction clamps, K-wires, dental picks, elevators, and laminar spreaders are all useful to help reduction. A medial side external fixator in a staged procedure can also help restore alignment and decrease soft tissue swelling (**Fig. 27**).
4. Intraoperative fluoroscopy should always include Broden and Harris views, which help to ensure anatomic reduction of the posterior facet and correction of varus malalignment and heel width.

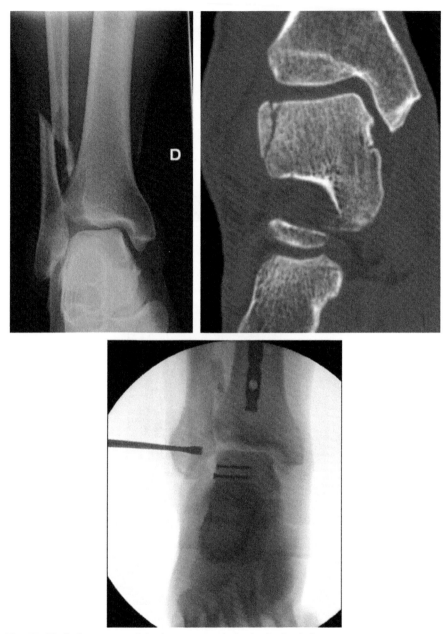

Fig. 17. Fibula fracture exploited to access a lateral talar body fracture.

5. Not all fractures have articular congruity. In some very comminuted Sanders type IV fractures, acute subtalar arthrodesis can be performed. However, it is important to combine it with an ORIF of the fracture before completing the fusion (**Fig. 28**).

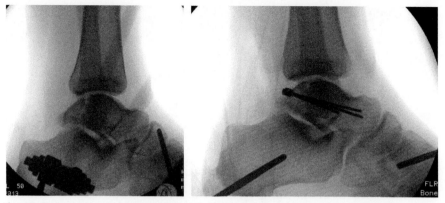

Fig. 18. Posterior medial approach and fixation of a very posterior talus fracture.

Fixation

1. Most fractures are fixed with a calcaneal plate associated with lag screws. In some cases, screw fixation alone is sufficient to maintain reduction. However, in most cases, the peripheral plate is necessary. Lag screws allow interfragmentary compression of the posterior facet. Stabilization of small displaced articular fragments using bioabsorbable pin fixation is useful to recreate a bone block for the posterior facet fragments.[7]
2. Isolated anterior process shear fractures should be addressed like Schatzker 2 tibial plateau fractures (**Fig. 29**). The articular fragment is disimpacted and rafting screws placed proximal to the joint. A buttress plate is added with or without additional bone graft.
3. Suture anchors are useful for additional fixation in tuberosity fractures. Isolated tuberosity fractures are generally treated using bicortical compression screws. A suture anchor can then be applied in the posterior tuberosity and weaved into

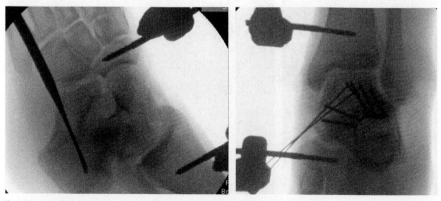

Fig. 19. Medial-based external fixator to help regain talar length.

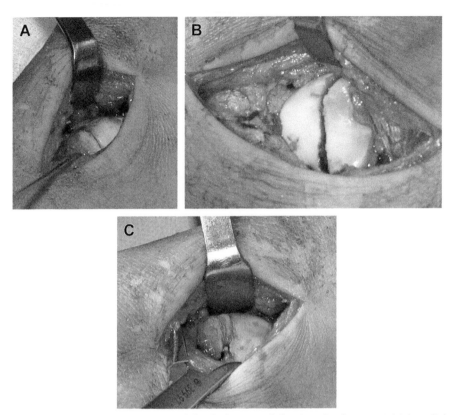

Fig. 20. Case showing the necessity of the dual approach for the talus fracture. Initial medial reduction (*A*) with incorrect lateral reduction (*B*). Correct medial reduction after identifying and reducing the comminuted medial fragment (*C*).

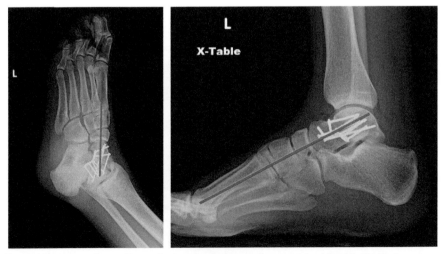

Fig. 21. Postoperative radiograph showing normal alignment (*red line*) in 2 views.

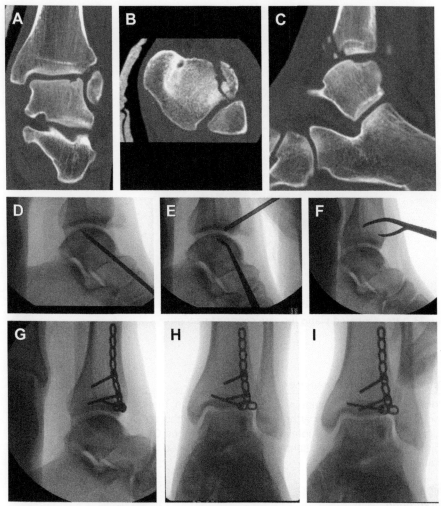

Fig. 22. Talar dome impaction fracture associated with a Chaput fragment fracture. (*A–C*) Retrograde drilling through a lateral wall cortical window was performed followed by disimpaction with the posterior surface of a curved curette. (*D–F*) Final result (*G–I*) of the talar fracture fixed and supported by injectable calcium sulfate.

the Achilles, slightly proximal to the tuberosity. This technique helps decrease distraction forces at the fracture site (**Fig. 30**).
4. Assess and treat peroneal tendon stability with a Freer before closing the flap. Peroneal tendon instability is common with calcaneal fractures. If the superior peroneal retinaculum is ruptured, the tendons can easily be subluxed using a Freer. The sheath can be repaired with a transosseous suture through a small lateral incision on the posterolateral border of the fibula (**Fig. 31**).

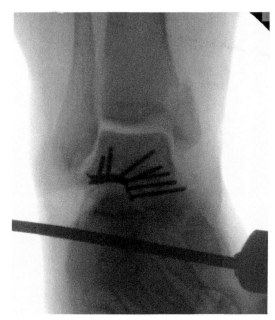

Fig. 23. Laterally based plates increase construct strength.

Complications and Management

Complications from calcaneus ORIF can be serious, therefore careful patient selection is essential. Subtalar arthritis is common, but this should not prevent surgeons from performing ORIF. Subtalar fusion after previous ORIF provides a better functional outcome than a subtalar fusion performed in an untreated calcaneal malunion.[8]

MIDFOOT FRACTURES
Background

Although several types of midfoot fracture exist (stress, avulsion) this the focus here is on high-energy fractures. Severe axial loading injuries to the midfoot often occur in polytraumatized patients and can go unnoticed. All foot swelling/ecchymosis must be investigated with appropriate imaging. The talonavicular joint is critical as the locking mechanism of the subtalar joint, and provides most of its mobility. Reconstructing this joint is of utmost importance. The cuboid, which was once thought to be protected by the calcaneus and fourth and fifth metatarsals, is essential for the lateral column. Restoring normal height makes it possible to recreate anatomic lateral column length and improves foot mechanics.

Preoperative Assessment

1. Preoperative assessment should be systematic, as described earlier.
2. Fracture dislocations should undergo closed reduction with or without external fixation. Dorsally extruded navicular can be particularly hard to reduce without external fixation. Temporary K-wire stabilization of the talonavicular joint is an option for grossly unstable joints.

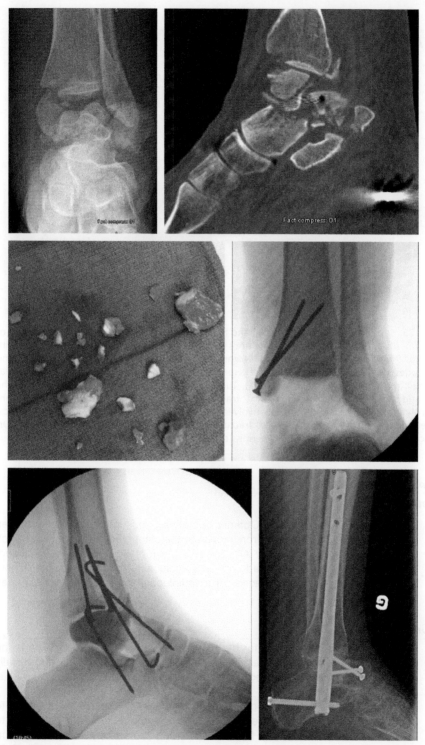

Fig. 24. Severely comminuted open talar fracture. Secondary infection treated with excision and definitive hind foot nail after infection was cured.

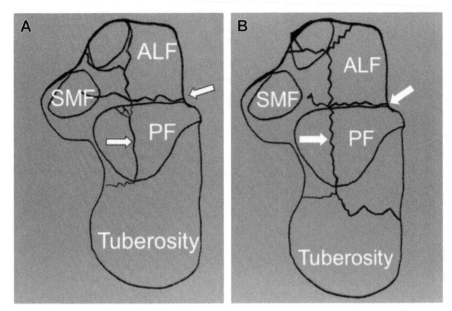

Fig. 25. Superior view of a tongue (*A*) and joint depression (*B*) fracture depicting the major fragments and the 2 primary fracture lines (*arrows*). Typical calcaneus fracture anatomy involves 5 fragments. The superomedial fragment (SMF) is called the constant fragment and includes the sustentaculum tali. The superolateral fragment involves an intra-articular aspect through the posterior facet (PF). The superolateral fragment can be divided in the PF and the lateral wall. The remaining 2 fragments are the tuberosity fragment and the anterolateral fragment (ALF), which involves the anterior process. (*From* Carr, JB. Surgical treatment of intra-articular calcaneal fractures: a review of small incision approaches. J Orthop Trauma 2005;19(2):110; with permission.)

Tips and Tricks

Patient positioning

1. Use multiple positional aids. Optimal operative exposure of the midfoot often requires going back and forth from supine to the plantigrade foot position, which is necessary to obtain quality AP views of the foot on fluoroscopic imaging. The affected leg is elevated on a radiolucent ramp or bump. Then, intraoperatively, the leg is placed on a radiolucent triangle to allow full knee flexion.

Surgical Approach

1. Longitudinal incisions are key for the navicular. The anteromedial incision is the workhorse for navicular fractures. It can be extended both proximally and distally as needed. This approach is necessary to get good visualization of plantar medial fragments.
2. Use fluoroscopy to locate cuboid incisions. Superficial anatomy can be hard to palpate in cuboid fractures. Ideally, the skin incision runs from the sinus tarsi to the base of the fourth and fifth metatarsals. Using fluoroscopy to locate the incision allows the surgeon to incise directly over and to the fracture (**Fig. 32**). Care should be taken to protect the sural nerve branches.

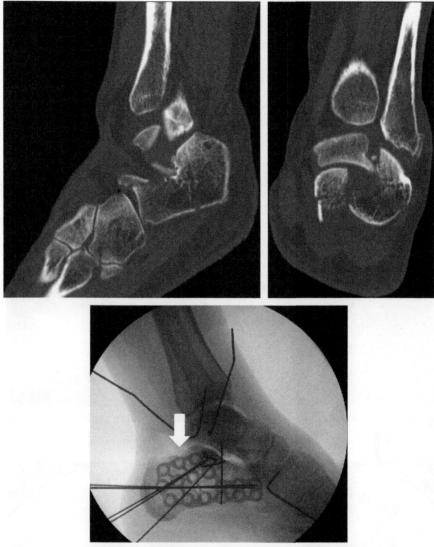

Fig. 26. Large tongue-type fragment did not enable visualization. It was osteotomized (*white arrow*) and reduced posteriorly, which allowed visualization of the posterior facet.

Reduction

1. Temporary external fixators are extremely useful. Medially, a pin is placed in the calcaneal tuberosity proximally and distally in the first metatarsal. Laterally, the proximal pin is placed in the calcaneal tuberosity and distally a small pin is placed in the fourth and fifth metatarsal necks, parallel to the joint (**Fig. 33**). This technique allows distraction and lengthening of both columns.

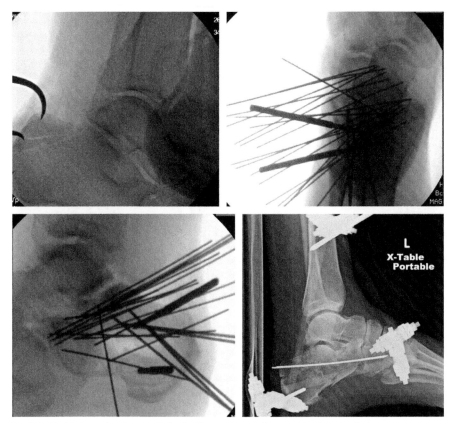

Fig. 27. Multiple reduction tools including external fixator, K-wires, and clamps.

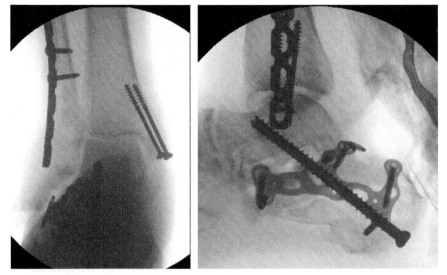

Fig. 28. Primary subtalar arthrodesis combined with ORIF in Sanders type IV fracture.

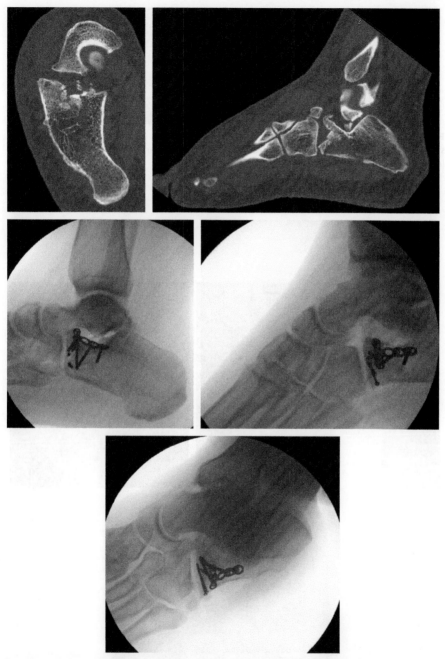

Fig. 29. Isolated anterior process shear fracture with marginal impaction. An anatomic reduction was obtained followed by grafting and fixation (combination of rafting screws and a buttress plate construct).

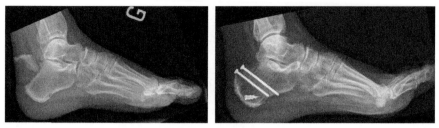

Fig. 30. Isolated displaced tuberosity fracture that is reduced with 2 bicortical screws and a suture anchor applied distal to the fracture in the posterior tuberosity to create an off-loading Achilles suture.

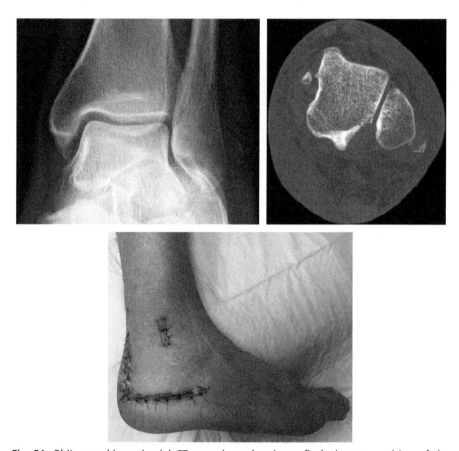

Fig. 31. Oblique ankle and axial CT scan views showing a flack sign, an avulsion of the posterolateral retinaculum with dislocated peroneal tendons. Foot showing the position of the incision for the retinaculum repair.

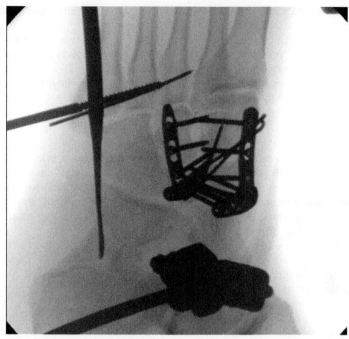

Fig. 32. A Freer is used to fluoroscopically locate the ideal incision for a cuboid ORIF.

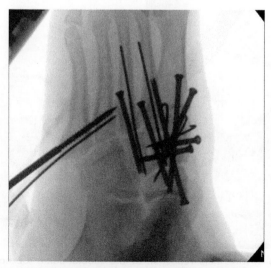

Fig. 33. Lateral external fixator into the fourth and fifth metatarsals.

These frames can also be left on after surgery to off-load and protect the fixation.

2. Provisional reduction and stabilization with K-wires is useful. As with most foot fractures, severely comminuted fractures can be rebuilt by independently fixing fragments to recreate the articular surface. Small-caliber K-wires can stabilize these fragments until rafting screws can be placed. Ultimately, these wires can be left as an adjunct to definitive fixation (**Fig. 34**).

Fixation

1. Fracture-specific plates are helpful. In some fracture patterns, specifically for the navicular, screw fixation is all that is required. However, in most cases, the degree of comminution requires plate stabilization to obtain adequate fixation. Many plates have been designed to specifically fit these oddly shaped bones. When specific plates are not available, standard mini–fragment plates can be adapted to fit most fractures (**Fig. 35**).

2. Spanning plates are sometimes necessary. With certain navicular fractures, severe comminution is impossible to address with screws. In these cases, supplemental fixation into the cuneiforms is necessary to prevent collapse. It is important not to span the talonavicular joint in order to preserve subtalar motion.

3. Use bone graft to fill voids. Then use more. The amount of axial loading to the cuboid and navicular required for fracture generally results in severe compression of trabecular bone. Once medial and lateral column lengths are restored, there is often a central void. Diligent filling using autograft or allograft helps reinforce fixation. A surprising amount of bone graft can be impacted into these fractures.

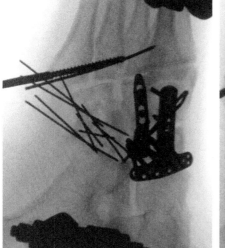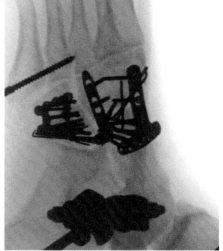

Fig. 34. Provisional K-wires help reduction of the cuboid. Some subchondral wires and fragment-specific cuboid plate are left for definitive fixation.

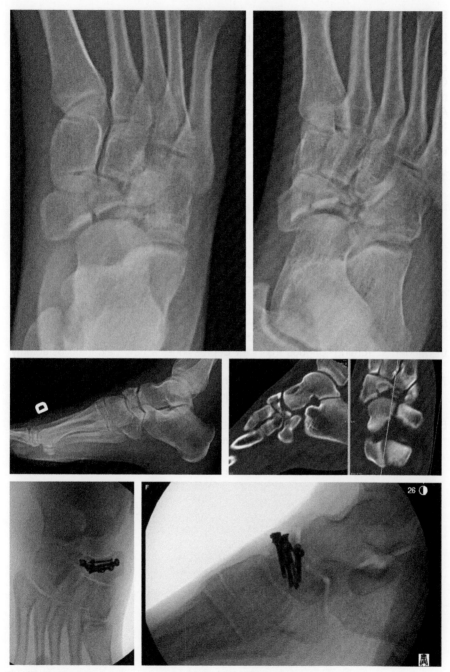

Fig. 35. Fragment-specific navicular plate with rafting screws and grafting.

SUMMARY

Foot and ankle fractures are not all benign injuries and are often associated with severe soft tissue injury. Although anatomic ORIF is the goal, the high-energy nature of some of these injuries makes them surgically challenging and technically complex. Good visualization and imaging are key to anatomic reduction. Using the techniques mentioned in this article should help surgeons achieve more positive outcomes. Although many techniques have been discussed in this article, they are only adjuncts to facilitate proper reduction and fixation.

REFERENCES

1. Tyler J, Van Heest BA, Paul M, et al. Injuries to the ankle syndesmosis. J Bone Joint Surg Am 2014;96(7):603–13.
2. Ricci WM, Tornetta P, Borrelli J Jr. Lag screw fixation of medial malleolar fractures: a biomechanical, radiographic, and clinical comparison of unicortical partially threaded lag screws and bicortical fully threaded lag screws. J Orthop Trauma 2012;26(10):602–6.
3. Gardner MJ, Demetrakopoulos D, Briggs SM, et al. Malreduction of the tibiofibular syndesmosis in ankle fractures. Foot Ankle Int 2006;27(10):788–92.
4. Borrelli J Jr, Leduc S, Gregush R, et al. Tricortical bone grafts for treatment of malaligned tibias and fibulas. Clin Orthop Relat Res 2009;467(4):1056–63.
5. Carr JB. Surgical treatment of intra-articular calcaneal fractures: a review of small incision approaches. J Orthop Trauma 2005;19(2):109–17.
6. Sander R. Turning tongues into joint depressions: a new calcaneal osteotomy. J Orthop Trauma 2012;26(3):193–6.
7. Min W, Munro M, Sanders R. Stabilization of displaced articular fragments in calcaneal fractures using bioabsorbable pin fixation: a technique guide. J Orthop Trauma 2010;24(12):770–4.
8. Radnay CS, Clare MP, Sanders RW. Subtalar fusion after displaced intra-articular calcaneal fractures: does initial operative treatment matter? J Bone Joint Surg Am 2009;91(3):541–6.

Current Swiss Techniques in Management of Lisfranc Injuries of the Foot

Fabian Krause, MD[a],*, Timo Schmid, MD[a], Martin Weber, MD[b]

KEYWORDS

- Lisfranc joint • Trauma • Open reduction and internal fixation • Technique

KEY POINTS

- The outcome after Lisfranc injuries correlates with anatomic and stable reduction.
- Appropriate reduction is achieved by open reduction and stable temporary screw or plate fixation.
- Symptom-free recovery is uncommon.
- In purely ligamentous Lisfranc injuries, open reduction and temporary fixation yield good results equal to primary arthrodesis, but maturation of a solid scar requires longer postoperative care.

INTRODUCTION: NATURE OF THE PROBLEM

The Lisfranc joint line, or tarsometatarsal joint (TMT) line, is a connection between the midfoot and forefoot. Being part of the midfoot arch, physiologic motion particularly in the central Lisfranc joint line, is highly restricted for load propulsion at push-off, whereas the lateral joints allow some dorsal motion for a more convenient rollover during gait. The metatarsal bases and the cuneiforms are dorsally based trapezoids in the coronal cross-section and build up a stable Roman arch that prevents plantar displacement of the metatarsal bases under load. Strong plantar and interosseous ligaments further stabilize the TMTs.

Lisfranc injuries are heterogeneous and range from high-energy midfoot injuries with severe disruption of the normal midfoot architecture, multiple associated injuries, and significant soft tissue injury to subtle subluxations and sprains that are frequently overlooked or misdiagnosed.[1,2] High-energy motor vehicle accidents are responsible for one-third to two-thirds of Lisfranc injuries, followed by crush injuries and falls from

The authors have nothing to disclose.

[a] Department of Orthopaedic Surgery, Inselspital, University of Berne, Freiburgstrasse, Berne 3010, Switzerland; [b] Department of Orthopaedic Surgery, Zieglerspital, University of Berne, Morillonstrasse 75, Berne 3007, Switzerland
* Corresponding author.
E-mail address: fabian.krause@insel.ch

ground level or height. Sports-related injuries are mostly provoked by axial loading of the plantar-flexed foot are increasing in number.[3]

Because of the stronger plantar ligaments, Lisfranc injuries usually lead to dorsal (and mostly lateral) dislocation of the TMT. A majority of Lisfranc injuries involve both disrupted ligaments and metatarsal, cuneiform, or cuboid fractures. There is also a small frequent subgroup of patients with a purely ligamentous injury.[1]

No correlation has been seen between the severity of the Lisfranc injury, the degree of diastasis, the pattern of displacement and final functional outcome.[4,5] Good and excellent results closely correlate, however, with anatomic reduction.[4,6] At present, open reduction and temporary internal fixation are recommended for Lisfranc fracture dislocation.[7,8] Closed reduction and percutaneous Kirschner wire (K-wire) or screw fixation have been advocated by several investigators in the past[9,10]; however, anatomic reduction, which is essential for optimal outcomes, is more reliably achieved and retained by open reduction and screw or plate fixation.[6,8,9,11,12] Furthermore, injuries exiting proximally through the intercuneiforms are less often missed by the open exposure. During surgery, a nonanatomic reduction of more than 2 mm in the representative anteroposterior, lateral, and oblique fluoroscopic views of the foot is inadequate.

Due to the multiplanar orientation of the small tarsometatarsal articular surfaces, closed anatomic reduction under fluoroscopic control is difficult. Furthermore, disrupted ligaments may prevent full reduction. Particularly in comminuted metatarsals, K-wires instead of screws or plates are more prone to loosening and migration, leading to fractures, loss of reduction, and often poor results.

As opposed to Lisfranc fracture dislocations with bony avulsions, inferior results have been reported for purely ligamentous Lisfranc injuries, if they are treated by open reduction and temporary internal fixation.[2,8,12]

A partial definitive arthrodesis of the first to third TMTs as a primary treatment of these patients was, therefore, suggested and supported by appropriate evidence.[2,6,12,13] Historically, arthrodesis of the TMT had been reserved as a salvage procedure after failed open reduction and temporary internal fixation, for a delayed or missed diagnosis, or for severely comminuted intra-articular fractures.[7,14,15]

One reason for failure of temporary fixation in the ligamentous injuries might be inappropriate postoperative management. The formation of a solid and reliable scar after ligamentous Lisfranc injuries likely takes much longer than fracture healing of the osseous Lisfranc injury or fusion of the primary Lisfranc arthrodesis.

The best surgical treatment, particularly for the ligamentous Lisfranc injuries, remains controversial. Despite appropriate surgical technique and postoperative management, symptom-free recovery is unusual, whereas midfoot collapse and arthritis occasionally require a conversion to a secondary arthrodesis.[9,16] This article outlines the current technique in the management of Lisfranc injuries and the corresponding postoperative outcome of the department of orthopedic surgery in a Swiss level I trauma center.

INDICATIONS/CONTRAINDICATION

Completely undisplaced and stable Lisfranc injuries, as determined by weight-bearing and/or stress radiographs, can be treated nonoperatively with immobilization and non–weight bearing for 6 to 8 weeks. Weight-bearing repeat radiographs are, however, recommended for any signs of interval displacement or diastasis, which would require surgical treatment.

For displaced and unstable injuries, current literature strongly supports surgical treatment because achieving and retaining anatomic reduction are prerequisites for a good outcome.

SURGICAL TECHNIQUE/PROCEDURE
Preoperative Planning

Severe Lisfranc injuries with wide displacement are accompanied by significant swelling, ecchymosis, deformity, and obvious radiographic signs. Subtle Lisfranc injuries without persistent subluxation are, however, often missed, predisposing to midfoot instability with chronic deformity and painful midfoot arthritis in the long-term. The plantar ecchymosis sign has been identified as an important clinical indicator for acute Lisfranc injuries and should prompt a high index of suspicion for tarsometatarsal instability (**Fig. 1**).

Clinical examination should also include looking for signs of an impending or already existing compartment syndrome that requires immediate fasciotomies of the midfoot compartments, particularly in high-energy injuries. Skin incisions for definitive fixation have to be taken into consideration when fasciotomy is performed. To avoid too proximal skin incisions or unnecessary distal extensions, incisions should be marked under fluoroscopic guidance. Despite respecting a minimum 4-cm skin bridge between skin incisions for fasciotomy, wound edge necrosis due to too much tension at secondary wound closure is commonly encountered, and a minimum skin bridge of more than 6 cm is, therefore, advised. Vessel loops applying moderate tension at the wound edges while the fasciotomies are open can prevent irreversible skin necrosis.

In crush injuries or severe displacement of the TMT, direct skin necrosis may occur. Prior to definitive surgery, severe displacements are aligned by closed reduction and retained by 1.6-mm K-wires to better enable subsidence of the soft tissue swelling. Open injuries are irrigated, débrided, and closed. Widely dehiscent wounds or soft tissue defects are closed by a vacuum dressing. Secondary soft tissue coverage, including skin grafts and myocutaneous or fasciocutaneous free flaps, are usually combined with the definitive surgery. Vascular compromise is a rare complication of tarsometatarsal dislocations.

Radiographic evaluation, including anteroposterior, lateral, and internal oblique radiographs of the foot, is frequently sufficient for decision making. A line drawn along every ray shows discontinuity or step-off even in subtle injuries. Mainly subtle Lisfranc injuries (up to 40%), however, are overlooked on initial radiographs, because they are non–weight bearing. Weight bearing radiographs are, therefore, obligatory to further evaluate the Lisfranc joint stability (**Fig. 2**) or abduction and adduction stress views under fluoroscopy, when acute pain and swelling has subsided after 1 or 2 weeks.

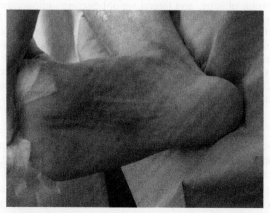

Fig. 1. The plantar ecchymosis sign.

A

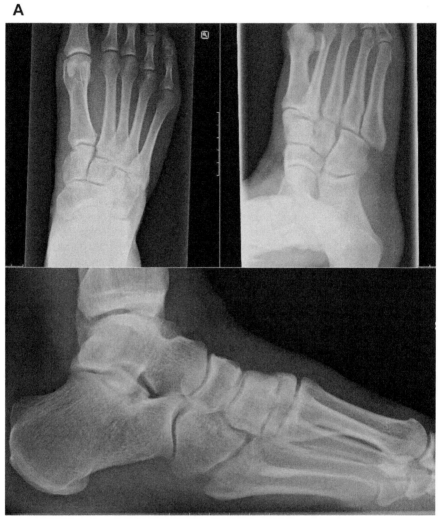

Fig. 2. Anteroposterior, oblique, and lateral weight-bearing radiographs of a 32-year-old male patient, taken in the emergency department. The patient had a fall from 4 m and sustained a subtle Lisfranc injury. (*A*) Note the bony irregularities between second metatarsal base and medial cuneiform. (*B*) In the CT scan of the same day, a plantar avulsion fracture of the second metatarsal base and a transverse fracture of the fourth metatarsal base were seen next to subtle signs of Lisfranc instability (*left side*) in comparison with contralateral (*right side*). (*C*) Five days after the trauma, the patient was able to bear weight on the injured foot, so that the Lisfranc instability is by far better visible.

Comparison views of the contralateral foot can add to confirming diagnosis. A CT scan allows assessment of concomitant fractures that are indicative of a Lisfranc injury. In purely ligamentous Lisfranc injury, a non–weight-bearing CT may not contribute additional information about the stability of a subtle injury (**Fig. 3**). In the acute injuries, an MRI or single-photon emission CT (SPECT) is of low importance for the evaluation of the stability and associated fractures. MRI has been reported, however, to have a high

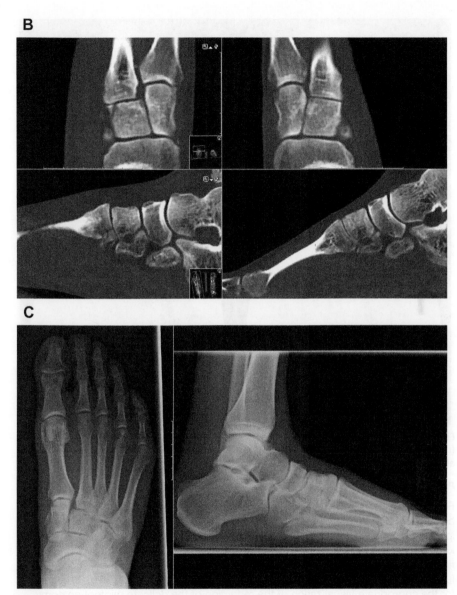

Fig. 2. (*continued*).

predictive value of Lisfranc injury by evaluation of the plantar component of the Lisfranc ligament.[17]

If for some reason surgery cannot be realized within 24 hours after trauma, the operation should be postponed for 4 to 7 days until swelling has appropriately subsided and skin wrinkles occur. Otherwise skin closure with too much tension can cause skin necrosis, wound breakdown, and deep infection. While awaiting surgery, patients should rest in bed with the foot elevated and immobilized in a non–weight-bearing lower leg cast. Patients with reliable reduction can be discharged home to reduce hospital cost.

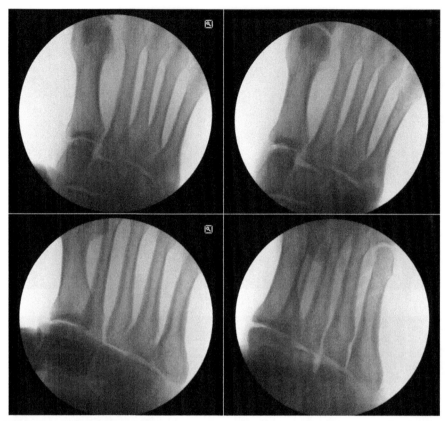

Fig. 3. Same patient as in Fig. 2. The corresponding views under fluoroscopy for the first (*upper row*) and second (*lower row*) intermetatarsal spaces without stress (*left*) and with abduction stress (*right*).

Preparation and Patient Positioning

For the open reduction and temporary internal fixation of Lisfranc injuries, the supine position on a radiolucent operation table is recommended. A bump underneath the ipsilateral thigh supports an upright position of the foot. The affected leg should be kept flexible in the hip and knee to allow easy and proper positioning of the foot for fluoroscopic visualization of all midfoot joints. A small and mobile fluoroscope is helpful (**Fig. 4**). A tourniquet with pressure ranging from 280 mm Hg to 350 mm Hg is useful for the appropriate visualization of the reduction of the delicate midfoot anatomy.

Depending on general health condition and accompanying injuries, all types of anesthesia can be applied. Intravenous second-generation cephalosporin antibiotics administered 30 minutes prior to surgery help reduce the infection rate and they are continued for 1 or 2 days postoperatively.

Surgical Approach

For definitive open reduction and internal fixation, a 4-cm to 6-cm longitudinal incision is centered between the first and second TMTs. To avoid unnecessary length and malposition of the incision, the incision is marked under anteroposterior fluoroscopy. This incision allows proper identification of the bony landmarks and anatomic reduction of the first and second TMTs. As needed in a majority of cases, the third TMT is

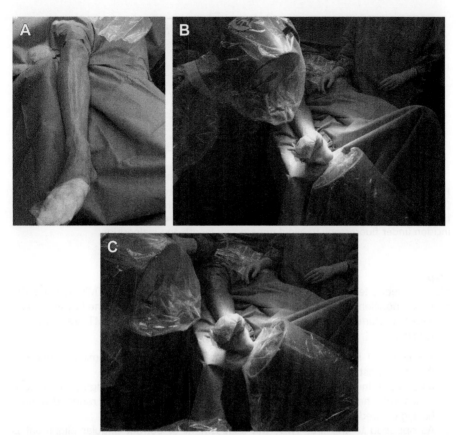

Fig. 4. The patient in supine position on a radiolucent operation table. (*A*) The affected leg should be kept flexible in the hip and knee to allow easy and proper positioning of the foot for fluoroscopic visualization of all midfoot joints. A small and mobile fluoroscope is helpful: positioning of the fluoroscope for the (*B*) first and (*C*) second intermetatarsal spaces.

reduced through the same incision, while the fixation screw is inserted by a 2-cm stab incision over the lateral base of the third metatarsal (**Fig. 5**).

It is recommended to extend the first incision rather than performing a second incision centered between the third and fourth rays, to avoid partial and full skin bridge necroses. If the second incision is inevitable for comminution of the third and/or lateral metatarsal bases or further midfoot fractures, a minimum distance of 4 cm between the 2 incisions and fully subsided soft tissues swelling is suggested. As opposed to the fasciotomy, this second incision is closed during the same surgery, and a minimum skin bridge of 6 cm is less important.

Crossing dorsal cutaneous branches of the superficial peroneal and saphenous nerves have to be respected when dissecting the subcutaneous tissue. The extensor hallucis longus tendon is retracted medially, whereas the extensor hallucis brevis tendon together with the neurovascular bundle is carefully retracted laterally.

Step 1
At this level, disruption of the dorsal TMT ligaments is usually obvious and the TMT and TMT are easy to identify. The second TMT is approximately 5 nm to 10 mm further proximal than first TMT (**Fig. 6**).

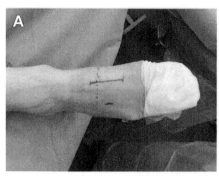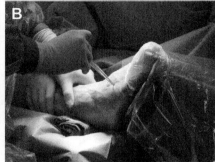

Fig. 5. A 4-cm to 6-cm longitudinal incision is marked between the first and second TMTs. (*A*) The third TMT is reduced through the same incision while the fixation screw is inserted by a 2-cm stab incision over the lateral base of the third metatarsal. (*B*) Positioning of the incision under fluoroscopy to avoid unnecessary length and malposition.

Step 2

Most surgeons tend to start the Lisfranc reduction at the second TMT because the recessed position of the second metatarsal base is thought to be the keystone. Advantages to starting and retaining Lisfranc reduction at the first TMT are, however, as follows:

1. The first TMT has the largest surface of all Lisfranc joints. Anatomic reduction is, therefore, best and easiest achieved and verified here.
2. Most often, the first TMT subluxes laterally beyond the lateral edge of the medial cuneiform. The second and third TMTs, however, cannot be fully reduced without having cleared the first metatarsal base.
3. As opposed to the first TMT, the assessment of correct angular alignment is more difficult at the second TMT because the surface is smaller, triangular, and frequently has comminuted plantar fragments.

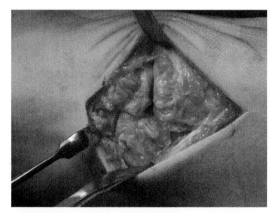

Fig. 6. Anatomy of unstable first and second TMTs (top = medial, bottom = lateral, and right = distal). These landmarks should visible for appropriate anatomic reduction. In this case, the capsule of the first TMT was detached and reflected, whereas the capsule of the second TMT was already torn.

4. Starting the temporary fixation at the large surface of the first TMT offers high initial mechanical stability during manipulation and reduction of the following second TMT.

Reduction in the axial and sagittal plane has to be judged carefully and verified with anteroposterior and lateral fluoroscopic views. To retain reduction until definitive fixation, a pointed reduction forceps or a small K-wire is helpful. For temporary internal fixation, a simple axial transarticular 3.5-mm, or in small feet a 2.7-mm, fully threaded, cortical screw is sufficient. Too much compression can cause a fracture of the dorsal metatarsal cortex and compromise the TMT cartilage over time. A notch technique could reduce the fracture risk but is unnecessary because the screws are removed after 3 months. In cases of a comminuted first metatarsal base, 2.0-mm screws are used to fix the reduced articular fragments while a bridging 2.7-mm or 2.4-mm dorsal plate retains anatomic alignment of the TMT.

Anatomic alignment and correct implant positioning are checked under fluoroscopy in the anteroposterior, lateral, and oblique planes to ensure malalignment does not interfere with anatomic reduction of the after TMT. A malalignment greater than 2 mm is not acceptable.

Step 3

After reduction and temporary fixation of the first TMT, the second and third TMTs usually need only subtle further adjustments. A pointed reduction forceps grasping the medial cuneiform from plantar and medial and the base of the second metatarsal from dorsal and lateral reduce the residual displacement of the second TMT under direct visualization (**Fig. 7**). Again, a retrograde axial transarticular 2.7-mm cortical screw, or in cases of metatarsal base comminution a bridging 2.7-mm or 2.4-mm dorsal plate, is used for temporary fixation. Correct alignment and implant positioning are checked under fluoroscopy (**Fig. 8**). The procedure is analaougously performed for the third ray, while the reduction forceps is placed dorsally and lateral onto the third metatarsal base and the screw is inserted via a stab incision slightly distal and lateral to the third metatarsal base. The Lisfranc screw that fixes the base of the second metatarsal to the medial cuneiform is, thereby, unnecessary in a majority of cases. Moving the first to third rays up and down in the sagittal plane assesses intercuneiforme stability.

Step 4

Rarely, there is residual instability of the fourth and fifth TMTs. The joint stabilizing ligaments of these TMT provide sufficient stability by ligamentotaxis. Fluoroscopic control of the lateral Lisfranc's stability is, however, obligatory. In approximately one-fifth of cases, particularly in high-energy injuries, closed reduction by a pointed reduction forceps, applied via stab incisions under fluoroscopic control, and temporary fixation by 1.6-mm K-wires, also under fluoroscopic control, are required of the fourth and fifth TMTs.

Step 5

Final anatomic alignment and appropriate implant positioning are verified under fluoroscopy (see **Fig. 7**). Tourniquet time ranges between 1 and a maximum of 2 hours depending on severity of the Lisfranc injury. The tourniquet is released and the wound is meticulously irrigated. After hemostasis, the longer incisions are closed in 2 layers with resorbable 3-0 Vicryl (Ethicon, Johnson & Johnson, Spreitenbach Mecial, Switzerland) subcutaneous sutures and 3-0 Vicryl rapid skin sutures, whereas resorbable skin sutures suffice for the stab incisions. A suction drain is unnecessary in a

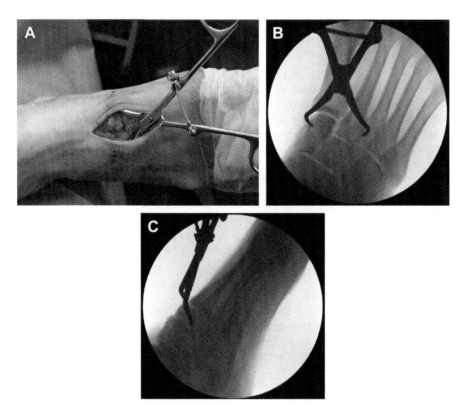

Fig. 7. (*A*) A pointed reduction forceps grasping the medial cuneiform from plantar and medial and the base of the second metatarsal from dorsal and lateral reduces the residual displacement of the second TMT under visualization by the eye and under fluoroscopy in the (*B*) anteroposterior and (*C*) lateral planes.

majority of cases. Next to the regular wound dressing, a noncircumferential plaster of Paris is applied in a plantigrade position.

Postoperative Care

Postoperatively, the foot is kept elevated in the plaster of Paris and the patient stays in hospital until wounds are dry. A closed non–weight-bearing plantigrade below-knee cast is applied at discharge. The patient is kept non–weight-bearing for 4 weeks.

At first follow-up 4 weeks postoperatively, the below-knee cast is changed, the wound controlled, and non–weight-bearing anteroposterior and lateral radiographs are taken. If everything is appropriate, 10-kg partial weight bearing in a new closed below-knee cast is allowed for another 4 weeks.

At second follow-up 8 weeks postoperatively, the below-knee cast is changed again, the wound controlled, and non–weight-bearing anteroposterior and lateral control radiographs are taken. K-wires of the fourth and fifth TMTs are removed between 6 and 8 weeks postoperatively. If everything seems ok, 20-kg partial weight bearing in a new closed below-knee cast is allowed for another 4 weeks, and the appointment for hardware removal 4 weeks later is fixed, including signature of informed consent for operation and anesthesia.

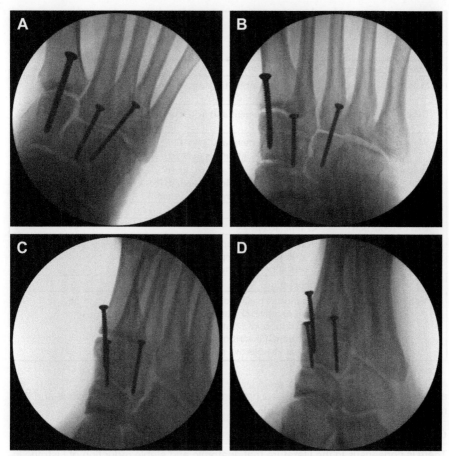

Fig. 8. Correct alignment and implant positioning are checked under fluoroscopy. (*A*) Alignment of first and second rays and of second and third rays in the coronal plane (*B*) and (*C*) first TMT and (*D*) second TMT in the sagittal plane are visualized by slight rotation.

At third follow-up 3 months postoperatively, the below-knee cast is removed, routine hardware removal is performed as a day-surgery procedure, and weight-bearing anteroposterior and lateral control radiographs are taken after hardware removal to confirm midfoot stability. The patient is kept 10 to 14 days 10 kg to 20 kg partial weight bearing until the new wounds have healed, followed by transition to full weight bearing within 2 to 4 weeks. An arch supporting custom-made orthotic is prescribed to be worn in a stable shoe or boot for 4 to 6 weeks, accompanied by physiotherapy, including strengthening and coordinative exercises.

At fourth follow-up, weight-bearing anteroposterior and lateral control radiographs are taken at 5 to 6 months postoperatively.

At fifth follow-up, weight-bearing anteroposterior and lateral control radiographs are taken at 1 year postoperatively; further follow-up is scheduled as needed.

Complications and Management

As **Table 1** shows, most immediate complications are related to wound issues. To avoid these complications, appropriate subsidence of the swelling prior to surgery

Table 1
Complications and management

		Incidence (%)
Immediate postoperative complications		
Superficial infection	Intravenous antibiotics, followed by oral antibiotics 5–10 d	15
Deep infection	Serial débridement and irrigation, antibiotics as needed	6
Wound breakdown	Serial débridement and irrigation, vacuum dressing, antibiotics as needed	3
Wound defect	Serial débridement and irrigation, vacuum dressing, antibiotics as needed, mesh graft Local or free flaps by plastic surgeons	3
Intermediate postoperative complications		
Loss of reduction	<2 mm: accept	31
Hardware failure	>2 mm: consider reoperation depending on time after surgery, compliance, age, activity level: refixation vs definitive arthrodesis	10
Long-term postoperative complications		
Midfoot arthritis	Diagnostic: plain radiographs, MRI or SPECT Nonoperative: (1) custom-made orthotic with arch support, (2) stiffened shoes with rocker bottom, (3) cortisone injections Operative: selective midfoot arthrodesis	36

and gentle intraoperative soft tissue handling is crucial. More complications and their management are presented in **Table 1**.

Outcomes

There is consensus in the literature that anatomic and stable reduction of Lisfranc injuries is a prerequisite for a good outcome.[4,7,8,15,17,18] Reported function and satisfaction scores, however, generally prove some ongoing discomfort without full recovery in a majority of cases. This is mainly caused by midfoot stiffness, loss of reduction, and arthritis in the long term (**Table 2**). Trends toward inferior outcome for purely ligamentous Lisfranc injuries treated with open reduction and internal temporary fixation have also been described.[2,6,18] Whether primary partial Lisfranc arthrodesis provides superior long-term outcome over temporary internal fixation remains controversial.[19]

As opposed to open reduction and screw fixation, dorsal plates can provide rigid fixation in Lisfranc injuries without further damage of the articular surfaces. In a cadaver model, the area of visible articular surface damage caused by a single 3.5-mm screw ranged from 2% to 5%.[20]

Another biomechanic cadaver study demonstrated that plates led to stiffer fixation and had less displacement than screws with static and cyclic loading.[21] No significant differences regarding functional outcome, pain, and midterm arthritis have been shown between transarticular screws and joint-sparing plates.[22] Long-term and prospective trials comparing transarticular screws versus dorsal plates are needed.

The authors' series compared the outcome of 29 purely ligamentous Lisfranc injuries of 135 Lisfranc injuries that were treated from 1998 to 2012 with open reduction, temporary internal fixation by transarticular screws to 29 osseous injuries, matched in age and gender and treated analogously.[19] The postoperative care followed the

Table 2
Outcome after Lisfranc injuries

	Kuo et al,[6] 2000	Perugia et al,[10] 2003	Rajapakse et al,[24] 2006	Rammelt et al,[25] 2008	Henning et al,[23] 2009	Ly and Coetzee,[18] 2006	Reinhardt et al,[13] 2012	Abbasian et al,[19] 2015
Patients	48	42	17	20	14	42	25	58
Follow-up (m)	52	58	43	37	24	43	42	96
Treatment	ORIF and screw	CRIF and screws	ORIF and screws	ORIF K-wires and screws	ORIF screws	ORIF or arthrodesis and screws	Primary partial arthrodesis	ORIF and screws
Arthritis	12	NA	NA	0	NA	15 of ORIF	3	9
Conversion to arthrodesis	6	NA	1	0	1	5 of ORIF	NA	2
Return to work	NA	NA	NA	NA	13	NA	NA	NA
AOFAS midfoot score[26]	80	81	78	81	NA	69 for ORIF 88 for arthrodesis	81	84
FFI[27]	NA	NA	NA	NA	NA	NA	NA	14.3
SF 36[28]	NA	NA	NA	NA	49	NA	52	56

Abbreviations: CRIF, closed reduction–internal fixation; m, months; NA, not applicable; ORIF, open reduction–internal fixation.

instructions (described previously), including a restricted weight bearing in below-knee cast for 3 months. The comparison revealed no significant differences in function and pain (American Orthopaedic Foot & Ankle Society [AOFAS] midfoot score, Foot Function Index [FFI] pain scale, 36-Item Short Form Health Survey [SF-36] physical and mental component, and Visual Analog Scale for Pain). Also, no substantial differences were seen comparing radiographic loss of reduction and arthritis between the groups at latest follow-up at 8 to 9 years. Only the FFI scale was significantly better in the ligamentous group.

The authors concluded, therefore, that open reduction and temporary internal fixation in ligamentous and osseous Lisfranc injuries led to appropriate medium-term outcome, equal to primary arthrodesis, when weight bearing was restricted in a below-knee cast for 3 months.[19] The long and conservative postoperative care was well accepted by the patients and led to less loss of reduction and midfoot arthritis.

To retain anatomic reduction after hardware removal in the ligamentous Lisfranc injuries, a strong scar formation has to build up prior to unprotected and full weight bearing. Appropriate scar formation likely takes longer than bony healing in osseous injuries and may require cast immobilization for 3 months with non–weight-bearing or partial weight bearing followed by an arch support for another 4 to 6 weeks.

Loss of reduction followed by midfoot arthritis was seen more frequently in series with shorter postoperative immobilization of only 6 to 8 weeks,[6,13,18] whereas superior maintenance of reduction was achieved after 3 months immobilization in other series.[23] An increase of stiffness or causalgia has not been noted with this prolonged immobilization.

The most important disadvantages of primary partial Lisfranc arthrodeses are a remarkable rate of 9% to 33% nonunions[8,13,18,23] and adjacent joint arthritis in 12% in the long term.[23]

SUMMARY

The outcome after Lisfranc injuries strongly correlates with an anatomic and stable reduction and is less dependent on the severity of the injury, the amount of initial diastasis, or pattern of displacement (see **Table 2**). The reduction is better achieved by open reduction and stable temporary screw or dorsal plate fixation than by closed reduction or K-wire fixation. Particularly in the ligamentous injuries, restricted weight bearing for 3 months followed by an arch support for another 4 to 6 weeks is recommended to build up a solid scar formation that prevents loss of reduction. A primary partial Lisfranc arthrodesis is, therefore, not the standard technique for ligamentous injuries.

REFERENCES

1. Chiodo CP, Myerson MS. Developments and advances in the diagnosis and treatment of injuries to the TMT joint. Orthop Clin North Am 2001;32(1):11–20.
2. Sheibani SS, Coetzee JC, Giveans MR, et al. Arthrodesis versus ORIF for Lisfranc fractures. Orthopedics 2012;35(6):e868–72.
3. Coker TP Jr, Arnold JA. Sports injuries to the foot and ankle. In: Jahss M, editor. Disorders of the foot. 1st edition. Philadelphia: WB Saunders; 1982. p. 1573.
4. Myerson MS, Fisher RT, Burgess AR, et al. Fracture dislocations of the TMT joints: end results correlated with pathology and treatment. Foot Ankle 1986;6(5):225–42.
5. Wilson DW. Injuries of the TMT joints. Etiology, classification and results of treatment. J Bone Joint Surg Br 1972;54(4):677–86.

6. Kuo RS, Tejwani NC, Digiovanni CW, et al. Outcome after open reduction and internal fixation of Lisfranc joint injuries. J Bone Joint Surg Am 2000;82(11): 1609–18.

7. Komenda GA, Myerson MS, Biddinger KR. Results of arthrodesis of the TMT joints after traumatic injury. J Bone Joint Surg Am 1996;78(11):1665–76.

8. Mulier T, Reynders P, Dereymaeker G, et al. Severe Lisfrancs injuries: primary arthrodesis or ORIF? Foot Ankle Int 2002;23(9):902–5.

9. Hardcastle PH, Reschauer R, Kutscha-Lissberg E, et al. Injuries to the TMT joint. J Bone Joint Surg Br 1982;64(3):349–56.

10. Perugia D, Basile A, Battaglia A. Fracture dislocations of Lisfranc's joint treated with closed reduction and percutaneous fixation. Int Orthop 2003;27:30–5.

11. Arntz CT, Veith RG, Hansen ST Jr. Fractures and fracture-dislocations of the TMT joint. J Bone Joint Surg Am 1988;70(2):173–81.

12. Trevino SG, Kodros S. Controversies in TMT injuries. Orthop Clin North Am 1995; 26(2):229–38.

13. Reinhardt KR, Oh LS, Schottel P, et al. Treatment of Lisfranc fracture-dislocations with primary partial arthrodesis. Foot Ankle Int 2012;33(1):50–6.

14. Mann RA, Prieskorn D, Sobel M. Mid-tarsal and TMT arthrodesis for primary degenerative osteoarthrosis or osteoarthrosis after trauma. J Bone Joint Surg Am 1996;78:1376–85.

15. Sangeorzan BJ. Outcome after open reduction and internal fixation of Lisfranc joint injuries. J Bone Joint Surg Am 2000;82(10):1609–18.

16. Buzzard BM, Briggs PJ. Surgical management of acute TMT fracture dislocation in the adult. Clin Orthop Relat Res 1998;(353):125–33.

17. Raikin SM, Elias I, Dheer S, et al. Prediction of midfoot injury in the subtle Lisfranc injury: comparison of magnetic resonance imaging with intraoperative findings. J Bone Joint Surg Am 2009;91:892–9.

18. Ly TV, Coetzee JC. Treatment of primarily ligamentous Lisfranc joint injuries: primary arthrodesis compared with open reduction and internal fixation. A prospective, randomized study. J Bone Joint Surg Am 2006;88(3):514–20.

19. Abbasian MR, Paradies F, Weber M, et al. Temporary internal fixation for ligamentous and osseous Lisfranc injuries: outcome and technical tip. Foot Ankle Int 2015;36(8):976–83.

20. Alberta FG, Aronow MS, Barrero M, et al. Ligamentous Lisfranc joint injuries: a biomechanical comparison of dorsal plate and transarticular screw fixation. Foot Ankle Int 2005;26(6):462–73.

21. Marks R, Parks B, Schon LC. Midfoot fusion technique for neuroarthropathic feet: biomechanical analysis and rationale. Foot Ankle Int 1998;19:507–10.

22. Hu SJ, Chang SM, Li XH, et al. Outcome comparison of Lisfranc injuries treated through dorsal plate fixation versus screw fixation. Acta Ortop Bras 2014;22: 315–20.

23. Henning JA, Jones CB, Sietsema DL, et al. Open reduction internal fixation versus primary arthrodesis for Lisfranc injuries: a prospective randomized study. Foot Ankle Int 2009;30(10):913–22.

24. Rajapakse B, Edwards A, Hong T. A single surgeon's experience of treatment of Lisfranc joint injuries. Injury 2006;37:914–21.

25. Rammelt S, Schneiders W, Schikore H, et al. Primary open reduction and fixation compared with delayed corrective arthrodesis in the treatment of tarsometatarsal (Lisfranc) fracture dislocation. J Bone Joint Surg Br 2008;90:1499–506.

26. Kitaoka HB, Alexander IJ, Adelaar RS, et al. Clinical rating systems for the ankle-hindfoot, midfoot, hallux, and lesser toes. Foot Ankle Int 1994;15(7):349–53.

27. Budiman-Mak E, Conrad KJ, Roach KE. The foot function index: a measure of foot pain and disability. J Clin Epidemiol 1991;44(6):561–70.
28. Carlsson AM. Assessment of chronic pain. I. Aspects of the reliability and validity of the visual analogue scale. Pain 1983;16(1):87–101.

Minimally Invasive Forefoot Surgery in France

 CrossMark

Tristan Meusnier, MD*, Prikesht Mukish, MD

KEYWORDS

- Forefoot surgery • Minimally invasive technique • Hallux valgus
- Metatarsal osteotomy • Arthrodesis • Morton neuroma

KEY POINTS

- Minimally invasive forefoot surgery is a modern concept that should be considered primarily as an efficient technical evolution of classical surgery.
- The improvement of the understanding of pathologies associated with a patient perpetual evolution of surgery facilitates the development of new concepts.
- The goal of minimally invasive surgery remains an improvement of results for the postoperative patient with functional optimization and early walking.

INTRODUCTION

For the past 25 years, forefoot surgery has been dramatically changing in France. The technical methods that concerned tendons, ligaments, and envelopes have spread to the bone itself. Before 1980, surgery was mostly practiced on the soft structures, consisting of mechanically stretching the distended elements located in the convexity and extending or cutting what was retracted into the concavities. Soft tissue interventions, such as the McBride and Peterson procedures, were used when the bone was healthy, and if the bone was sick, articular sacrifices, bone resections (as the base of the first phalanx [P1] of the hallux), or complex and stiffness bone surgeries, including the inferior Schnepp procedure, were then realized.

Pathophysiologically, the medial projection in hallux valgus is primarily related to the angulation of the first metatarsal (M1) (metatarsus varus), with the proximal phalanx of the hallux (P1) associated with the phenomena of pronation and elevatus. Efforts seeking to reduce the deformity by tensioning the soft parts is doomed to failure. The first in France to popularize mechanical logic of M1 relaxation osteotomy was Patrice Diebold[1]: he brought back from the United States, in the 1980s, the "V"distal epiphyseo-metaphyseal osteotomy of the first metatarsal called "chevron." Shortly before, he had started the first phalangeal osteotomies.

The authors have nothing to disclose.
Foot and Ankle Surgery Center, Clinique Saint Charles, 25 rue de Flesselles, Lyon 69001, France
* Corresponding author.
E-mail address: drmeusnier@wanadoo.fr

Foot Ankle Clin N Am 21 (2016) 351–365
http://dx.doi.org/10.1016/j.fcl.2016.01.007   foot.theclinics.com
1083-7515/16/$ – see front matter © 2016 Elsevier Inc. All rights reserved.

Later, in the early 1990s, Samuel Barouk discussed in France the diaphyseal osteotomy of the first metatarsal (M1), called scarf.[2] This surgery was widely circulated in France and became the gold standard for correction of hallux valgus.

Gradually, surgical methods were increasingly developed with improvement of surgical technique itself even with respect for the bone environment and for the neighboring soft tissues on the bigger toe and on the lateral rays.[3]

Minimally invasive surgery and the use of a mini skin incision should not be confused. The length of the scar can certainly be important in terms of esthetics for the patient, but it does not define the quality of surgery realized in depth. For us, the real minimally invasive surgery is the one that respects the profound anatomic elements (vascularization, muscles, tendons, ligaments, capsule, bones) and that provides sufficient visibility to safely realize the surgical gesture, without abusing the skin, where nearly all infections originate. Furthermore, the quantity of material of osteosynthesis and its volume also participate in this concept of minimally invasive surgery.

Rather than writing long descriptive phrases, we describe our minimally invasive surgical techniques in the surgery of the forefoot.

HALLUX VALGUS: MAESTRO'S MODIFIED SCARF OSTEOTOMY OF THE FIRST METATARSAL, OUR TECHNIQUE

Scarf osteotomy of the first metatarsal bone to correct hallux valgus deformity has benefited from a number of improvements over the past 2 decades, most notably regarding the internal fixation method.[4–10] Maestro suggested eliminating the proximal screw by locking the 2 fragments distally: a notch was created via a medial extension of the cephalic part of the osteotomy, the plantar fragment was displaced laterally, and the distal end of the proximal fragment was then fit into the notch (secondary cut and interlocking joint technique). To further develop this concept and to increase the potential range of translation, an original technique was developed involving distal locking without shortening and proximal stabilization by impaction of a cortical-cancellous bone graft taken from the medial overhanging edge of the proximal fragment. It requires no screws for internal fixation.

A short medial incision is made next to the metatarsophalangeal articulation of the first ray. Careful hemostasis of blood vessels is performed to reduce postoperative bleeding and to reduce hemorrhagic complications and especially reduce postoperative edema. The dissection is continued until the joint capsule. It is realized that a neurolysis of the dorsal sensory nerve in the plane of the joint capsule would lessen suffering and avoid its suture during the capsular closure (**Fig. 1**).

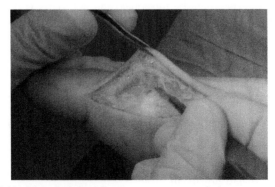

Fig. 1. Skin medial incision and dorsal sensory nerve neurolysis.

The joint capsule is opened, maintaining a periosteal and capsular flap sectioned at the metatarsal level and left attached to the phalanx to allow postoperative creation of a neo-ligament strengthening the medial plane, which fails in this pathology (**Fig. 2**).

The medial exostosis is removed with an oscillating saw. Then, to avoid an additional commisural incision and stay in the concept of minimally invasive surgery, the bed of the sesamoids is released to achieve an endo-articular passing under the first metatarsal head and taking care to avoid injury to the lateral ligament, thus risking a postoperative hallux varus (**Fig. 3**).

The osteotomy areas are released at minimum, taking care to leave the head of the first metatarsal well vascularized with its plantar pedicle and its dorsal vascularization. It reduces the risk of bone nonunion and scar fibrosis, which is responsible for postoperative stiffness (**Fig. 4**).

Making a short scarf modified Maestro osteotomy allows for translation, shortening, lowering, or derotation on demand. The embedding of the bone is possible through the realization of notches.

An impaction of the osteotomy area makes it a self-stable reduction. No forceps are required to maintain the reduction, limiting aggression of the soft tissues locally. With adequate stability and good impaction of the bone, it is not necessary to provide additional internal fixation. A distal osteosynthesis can be achieved by a small screw. Excess medial bone is cut with the saw, turned, and impacted in the proximal metaphyseal of M1, thus preserving bone mass and stabilizing the realized reduction (**Figs. 5** and **6**).

A release of the abductor of the great toe, which is just in the plantar part of the incision, is performed to soften support tissues and improve walking (**Fig. 7**).

A medial ligament reinforcement is produced with the capsule-periosteal flap and after that capsule's suture is made (**Fig. 8**). We think that the best tensioning position of the new medial ligament is when the great toe is in a plantar position (approximately 20°) and with a small valgus of the first phalanx (approximately 5°).

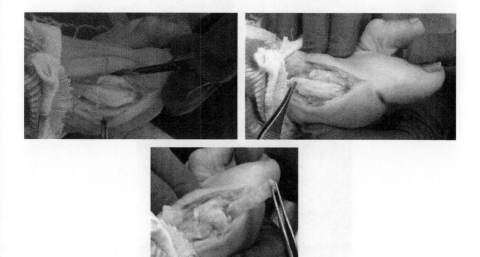

Fig. 2. Medial capsular opening by maintaining a medial neo-ligament inserted on the phalanx.

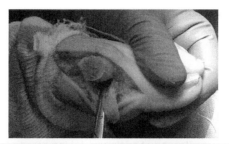

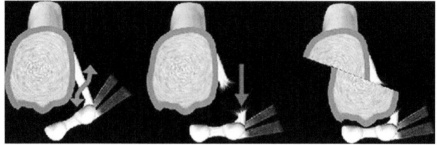

Fig. 3. Endo-articular release of the bed of the sesamoid. This release permits the translation of the first metatarsal osteotomy.

An osteotomy of the first phalanx is then realized, if it is needed, to shorten or to straighten or to act against the pronation of the great toe. In this case, there is a place for percutaneous surgery[11] for us and for French surgeons. A complementary osteosynthesis can be used or not.

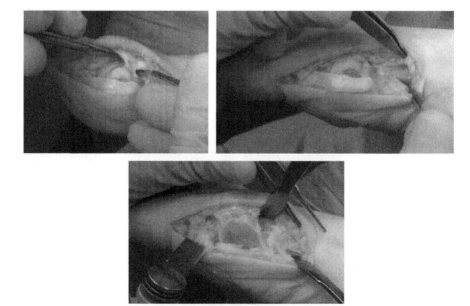

Fig. 4. Minimally invasive liberation of the first metatarsal for scarf osteotomy. The dorsal and plantar vascularization are preserved and the exposure of the metatarsal is minimal for less traumatism.

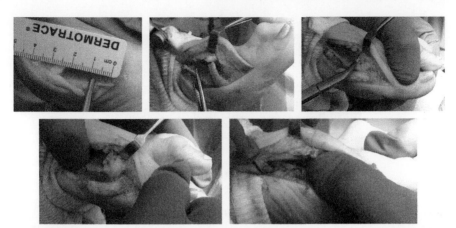

Fig. 5. Maestro stable scarf osteotomy. A short scarf osteotomy is made. Proximal and distal notches are created. The translation of the scarf osteotomy is made with an impaction of the bone by using the notches.

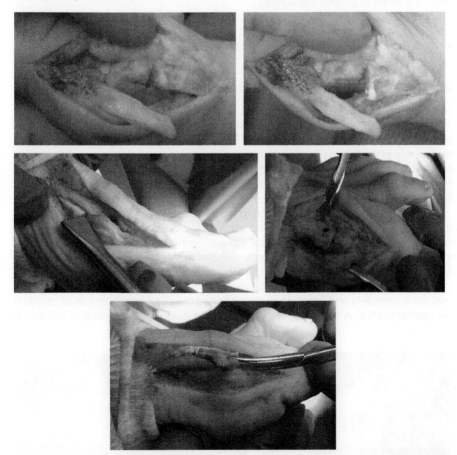

Fig. 6. Maestro stable scarf osteotomy. After the impaction, a resection of the medial bone is done with a bone grafting inside the proximal metaphyseal metatarsal to conserve the bone and to extend the auto-stability. A screw fixation in the head of the first metatarsal can also be used.

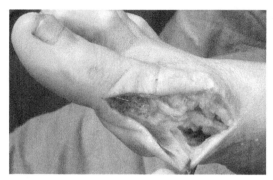

Fig. 7. Release of the abductor longus of the great toe.

The closure is performed intradermally. In our practice, we make a radiograph in the operating room to control the surgery.

A well-positioned dressing on the toe is left in place for 3 weeks. Postoperative suitable footwear with appropriate support is precontoured for faster functional recovery with postoperative physiotherapy recommended (**Figs. 9** and **10**).

OSTEOTOMY OF THE LATERAL METATARSALS

The Weil osteotomy was performed by L.S. Weil (Chicago) in 1985. It is an oblique distal metatarsal osteotomy that provides longitudinal decompression but can also provide a medial or lateral translation.[12–16] In 1992, Weil came to Bordeaux to attend the first day of the French scarf, and during a live surgery, he practiced the first case of the Weil osteotomy in Europe. Since then, this technique has been widely studied. The main problem with this technique is the stiffness of the metatarsophalangeal plantar flexion and the lowering of the metatarsal head.

To reduce the risk of stiffness related to the wide opening of the joint capsule and to limit the lowering of the metatarsal head, we have developed another cervical osteotomy called "OCRA."[17] To avoid many vertical approaches in intermetatarsal spaces, we carry a transverse dorsal approach centered on the metatarsal heads that can be extended, according to the preoperative planning, to the desired metatarsal.

A shortening osteotomy of the metatarsal with 2 saw cuts is performed. The proximal cut is complete and interests all the bone and the distal osteotomy must maintain the plantar cortex. A corresponding preoperative planning bone puck is extracted.

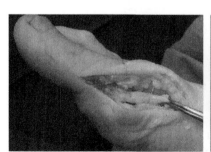
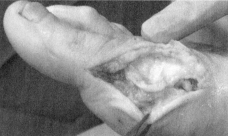

Fig. 8. Medial neo-ligament and capsule clothing.

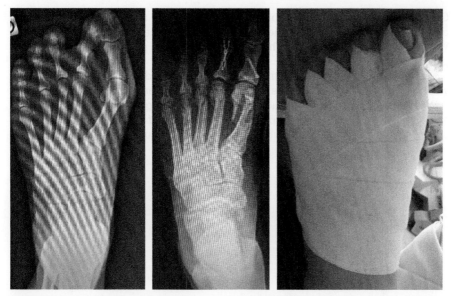

Fig. 9. Correction of hallux valgus with a scarf modified Maestro osteotomy with one screw for fixation (this patient also had an interphalangeal arthrodesis of the second toe and percutaneous osteotomies of the second, third, and fourth metatarsal). Note the postoperative dressing with well-positioned toe.

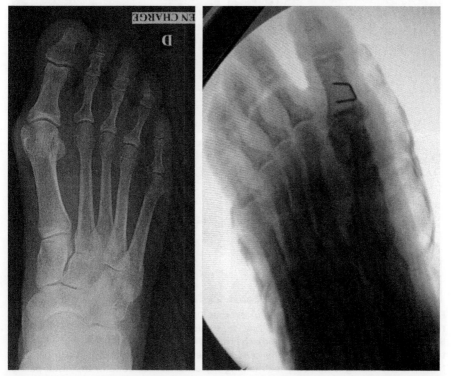

Fig. 10. Correction of hallux valgus with a scarf modified Maestro osteotomy without screw fixation.

Compression is realized and stabilization is achieved by a breakable (2-mm) screw and this stabilization is increased by the plantar cortical preservation, unlike the Weil osteotomy (**Figs. 11–12**). The conservation of the plantar cortex allows less plantar flexion of the metatarsal.

Moreover, the joint head of the metatarsal is not exposed to achieve the osteotomy, which reduces the risk of stiffness. This is truly an extra-articular osteotomy.

We also think that there is a place in percutaneous surgery for the lateral metatarsals.[18,19] If there is not much decompression needed and if there is no problem with subluxation of the metatarsophalangeal joint, we use percutaneous techniques (distal

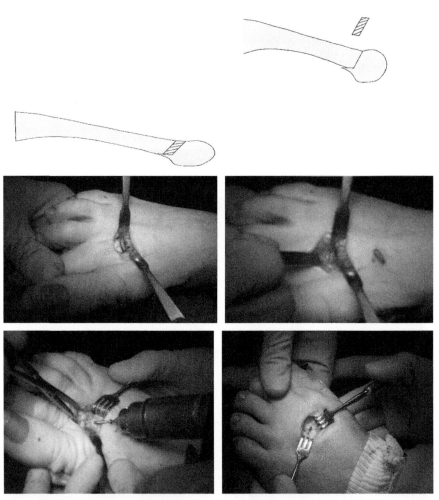

Fig. 11. The OCRA metatarsal technique. Top row: Osteotomy of the metatarsal maintaining the plantar distal cortical, which allows shortening, more stability, and less lowering. Bottom row: A transversal dorsal approach is made. A small exposure after passing between the extensor tendons is realized. The head and the metaphysis are exposed without luxation. The shortening is made by maintaining a plantar cortica bone in the distal part of the osteotomy. After that, compression is made and then stabilization with a breakable 2-mm screw is recommended.

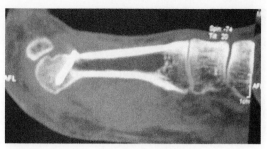

Fig. 12. Scan postoperative view of an OCRA osteotomy.

metatarsal minimally invasive osteotomy, DICMO [distal intra capsular metatarsal osteotomy]). In these cases, the postoperative closure is very important and is always done by the surgeon himself (see **Fig. 9**).

The Akin osteotomy of the first phalanx can be performed with classical surgery, but in France, some of the surgeons use percutaneous surgery. It can be fixed (with a screw or a staple) or not.

We are actually in a new era of hybrid surgery in France, achieved by the combination of conventional and percutaneous operative techniques.

ARTHRODESIS OF THE METATARSOPHALANGEAL ARTICULATION OF THE GREAT TOE

The first metatarsal joint fusion is indicated in cases of arthritis, hallux valgus over 50°, reoccurrence of hallux valgus after conservative treatment, and for resolving a hallux valgus with neurologic disease. The hallux valgus associated with a posterior tibial tendon tendinosis or a flat foot is also an indication of the first metatarsophalangeal articulation fusion. It will stiffen and stabilize the first column.

The aim of the arthrodesis is to fuse the first metatarsophalangeal articulation in a functional position. This position is quite hard to define in valgus or dorsiflexion. The residual valgus deformity must be corrected to avoid a conflict between the second toe and the great toe. This conflict can cause discomfort and an ingrown nail.

The dorsiflexion must allow for shoes with a 3-cm heel for women and 2 cm for men. It must also allow, when walking barefoot, a simultaneous rest under the great toe, the first metatarsal head, and the heel.

The functional position is different when talking about men, women, and flat or claw foot. The flat foot needs a very low dorsiflexion, whereas the claw foot needs more dorsiflexion than a normal foot, avoiding the spontaneous flexion of the interphalangeal joint (**Fig. 13**).

The hardware must permit the different positioning. The plates are convenient but are quite strict regarding to their positioning. Regarding this consideration, we chose to fix our arthrodesis with soft pure titanium nail. This nail was an evolution of Georges Gauthier's staple, which was modified by the group "pied innovation."

To push the concept of minimally invasive surgery, we use a system of elastic intramedullary nailing associated with a back staple. This system is easy to use, not constrained to any position, and is not invasive locally because it

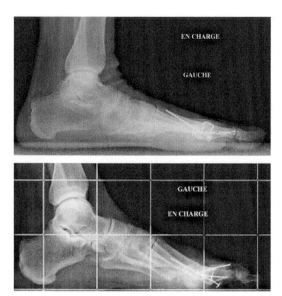

Fig. 13. Different positions for the arthrodesis of the metatarsophalangeal articulation of the great toe. Top: A flat foot needs a very low dorsal flexion. Bottom: A claw foot needs a more important dorsal flexion.

takes up very little space. Furthermore, it allows a good compression of the fusion area.

The principle is adaptable to every case in terms of morphology and bone quality. It was inspired by the elastic stable intramedullary nailing[20,21] (**Fig. 14**). If it is a soft fixation, the joint resection must be flat, avoiding the curved resection. The flat resection gives a spontaneous stability.

The fixation is a 3-step technique that gives progressive stability and compression. The 2 introductory nail holes are quite plantar. The first nail is introduced from the metatarsal to the phalanx. The second nail is driven from the phalanx to the metatarsal. The dorsal staple controls the rotation (**Fig. 15**). The fusion

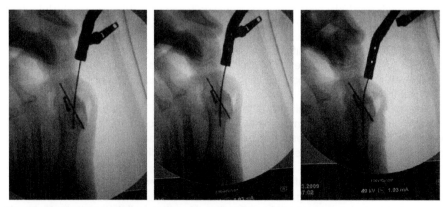

Fig. 14. Elastic intramedullary nailing for arthrodesis of the great toe.

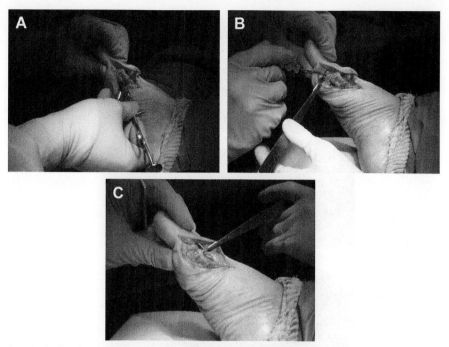

Fig. 15. Arthrodesis of the great toe with elastic intramedullary system. (*A*) The first nail is introduced from the metatarse to the phalanx. (*B*) The second nail is driven from the phalanx to the metatarse. (*C*) The dorsal staple controls the rotation.

rate is more than 98% after 45 days. It is a very convenient and reproducible technique.[22–26]

The bone resection is performed with a manual rongeur to avoid bone burning. It is a strict ambulatory procedure with immediate weight bearing with flat stiff shoes. The plantar shoe plate is removed after 21 days to allow a free step (**Fig. 16**). After 1 month, driving a car is permitted and after 45 days a progressive return to all activity is allowed.

MORTON DISEASE

When conservative medical treatment is worn out, surgeons have a few options regarding how to treat the neuroma.

One school of thought is to remove the offending ligaments, which then decompresses the nerve while keeping it intact. It can be similar to surgery of the hand for decompression of the median nerve. This surgery can be performed with a dorsal incision or a commissural incision. It also can be performed with percutaneous or endoscopic surgery.

Another school of thought is to remove the nerve that has been affected by the Morton neuroma entirely (**Fig. 17**). With the damaged nerve tissue removed, the neuroma is less likely to recur, and the mechanical stresses on the foot are not increased. Most surgeons are proponents of this latter theory and remove the affected nerve, although some patients may require a different method.[27–29]

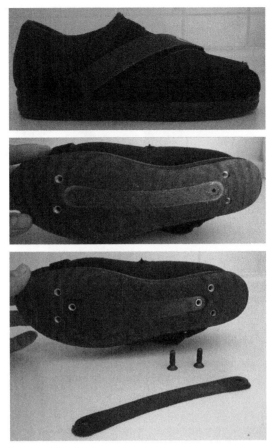

Fig. 16. Postoperative modular shoes.

We actually remove the nerve when the examination shows a consequent neuroma and perform a neurolysis when the neuroma is small. It is also important to consider the choice of the patient.

SUMMARY

Minimally invasive forefoot surgery is a modern concept that should be considered primarily as an efficient technical evolution of classical surgery.

The improvement of the understanding of pathologies associated with a patient perpetual evolution of surgery facilitates the development of new concepts. Whether in terms of pure surgery (eg, reduction in the size of skin incisions, respect for soft tissue, respect of the vascularization, preservation of the bone, improving existing osteotomies) or in terms of equipment of osteosynthesis used (eg, improved materials, reducing the quantity and the volume of material used), the goal of minimally invasive surgery remains an improvement for postoperative patients in results with functional optimization and early walking.

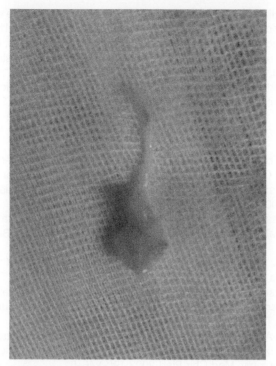

Fig. 17. Extraction of Morton neuroma.

Forefoot surgery has yet to be explored and developed. Many French and European research groups are currently in place, under the leadership of scientific societies, to develop and analyze these new concepts.

REFERENCES

1. Diebold PF. Ostéotomie distale épiphyso-métaphysaire en chevron dans l'hallux valgus. Med Chir Pied 1994;10:102–7.

2. Barouk LS. Scarf osteotomy of the first metatarsal in the treatment of hallux valgus. Foot Dis 1995;2:35–48.

3. Laffenêtre O, Golano P, GRECMIP. Introduction to foot and ankle minimally invasive surgery. E-mémoires de l'Académie Nationale de Chirurgie 2010;9(1):52–60.

4. Leemrijse T, Maestro M, Tribak K, et al. Scarf osteotomy without internal fixation to correct hallux valgus. Orthop Traumatol Surg Res 2012;98(8):921–7.

5. Maestro M. Scarf osteotomy without screw fixation. Interactive Surg 2007;2(1): 12–6.

6. Gonzalez JF, Rochwerger A, Curvale G, et al. 287 osteotomies de Scarf pour hallux valgus: l'ostéosynthèse est-elle indispensable? Rev Chir Orthop 2008. http://dx.doi.org/10.1016/S0035-1040(07)79627-7.

7. Borrelli AH, Weil LS. Modified scarf bunionectomy: our experience in more than 1000 cases. J Foot Surg 1991;30:609.

8. Valtin B. Quelle osteotomie pour quel hallux valgus ? Table ronde sur les « ostéotomies de premier métatarsien dans le traitement chirurgical de l'hallux valgus ». Med Chir Pied 1994;10:121–8. Expansion scientifique française, Paris.

9. Wagner A, Fuhrmann B, Abramoski I. Early results of scarf osteotomies using differentiated therapy of hallux valgus. Foot Ankle Surg 2000;6:105–12.

10. Weil LS. Scarf osteotomy for correction of hallux valgus. Historical perspective, surgical technique and results [review]. Foot Ankle Clin 2000;5(3):559–80.

11. Ghorbani A, Bauer T. Osteotomie de la phallange proximale de l'hallux. In: Chirurgie mini-invasive et percutanée du pied. Sauramps Medical; 2009. p. 121–6.

12. Barouk LS. L'ostéotomie cervico-céphalique de Weil dans les métatarsalgies médianes. Med Chir Pied 1994;1:23–33. Expansion scientifique française, Paris.

13. Hart R, Janeeck M, Bucek P. The Weil osteotomy in metatarsalgia. Z Orthop Ihre Grenzgeb 2003;141(5):590–4 [in German].

14. Jarde O, Hussenot D, Vimont E, et al. L'ostéotomie cervico-capitale de Weil dans les métatarsalgies médianes, étude de 70 cas. Acta Orthop Belg 2001;67(2): 139–48.

15. Melamed EA, Shon LC, Myerson MS, et al. Two modifications of the Weil osteotomy: analysis on sawbone. Foot Ankle Int 2002;25(9):400–5.

16. Henry J, Besse JL, Fessy MH. Distal oeteotomy of the lateral metatarsals: a series of 72 cases comparing the Weil osteotomy and the DMMO percutaneous osteotomy. Orthop Traumatol Surg Res 2011;97(6 suppl):S57–65.

17. Benichou M, Augoyard M, Leemrisje T, et al. A new central metatarsal osteotomy: the cervical axial shortening osteotomy. A comparative geometric approach with the Weil osteotomy. Med Chir Pied 2003;19(2):46–51.

18. Coillard JY. Distal metatarsal minimally invasive osteotomy (DMMO). In: Chirurgie Mini-Invasive et Percutané du pied. Sauramps Medical, GRECMIP; 2009. p. 127–34.

19. De Prado M, Ripoll PL, Golano P, editors. Cirugia percutanea del pie. Barcelona (Spain): Masson; 2003. p. 165–74. Part 4 Capitulo 10, metatarsalgias.

20. Ligier JN, Metaizeau JP, Prévot J, et al. Elastic stable intramedullary pinning of long bone shaft fractures in children. Z Kinderchir 1985;40(4):209–12.

21. Lascombes P, Prevot J, Ligier JN, et al. Elastic stable intramedullary nailing in forearm shaft fractures in children: 85 cases. J Pediatr Orthop 1990;10(2): 167–71.

22. Roukis TS, Meusnier T, Augoyard M. Nonunion rate of first metatarsal-phalangeal joint arthrodesis for end-stage hallux rigidus with crossed titanium flexible intramedullary nails and dorsal static staple with immediate weight-bearing. J Foot Ankle Surg 2012;51(3):308–11.

23. Roukis TS, Meusnier T, Augoyard M. Nonunion rate of first metatarsal-phalangeal joint arthrodesis with crossed titanium flexible intramedullary nails and a dorsal static staple with immediate weightbearing. J Foot Ankle Surg 2012;51(2):191–4.

24. Roukis TS, Meusnier T, Augoyard M. Arthrodesis of the first metatarsal-phalangeal joint with flexible, ridged titanium intramedullary nails alone or supplemented with static staples and immediate weight bearing: a consecutive series of 148 procedures. Foot Ankle Spec 2012;5(1):12–6.

25. Mahadevan D, Korim MT, Ghosh A, et al. First metatarsophalangeal joint arthrodesis—Do joint configuration and preparation technique matter? J Foot Ankle Surg 2015;21(2):103–7.

26. Roukis TS, Meusnier T, Augoyard M. Incidence of nonunion of first metatarsophalangeal joint arthrodesis for severe hallux valgus using crossed, flexible titanium

intramedullary nails and a dorsal static staple with immediate weightbearing in female patients. J Foot Ankle Surg 2012;51(4):433–6.

27. Bauer T, Gaumetou E, Klouche S, et al. Metatarsalgia and Morton's disease: comparison of outcomes between open procedure and neurectomy versus percutaneous metatarsal osteotomies and ligament release with a minimum of 2 years of follow up. J Foot Ankle Surg 2015;54(3):373–7.

28. Villas C, Florez B, Alfonso M. Neurectomy versus neurolysis for Morton's neuroma. Foot Ankle Int 2008;29(6):578–80.

29. Barrett SL. Endoscopic nerve decompression [review]. Clin Podiatr Med Surg 2006;23(3):579–95.

State-of-the-Art in Ankle Fracture Management in Chile

Cristián A. Ortiz, MD*, Pablo Wagner, MD, Emilio Wagner, MD

KEYWORDS

- Ankle fracture • Deltoid ligament rupture • Syndesmotic instability
- Lateral malleolar fracture • Ankle fracture rehabilitation • State-of-the-art • Review

KEY POINTS

- Fibular displacement is not an independent factor to decide surgical intervention.
- Joint congruity and medial stability are the key points when deciding between surgical versus nonsurgical treatment.
- Posterior malleolus fractures should be operated with a low threshold.
- Percutaneous screws, posteromedial plates, or posterior plates are the treatment options depending on the fracture type.
- For surgical or nonsurgical isolated lateral malleolar fractures, weight bearing is permitted as tolerated on postoperative day 1; with all other fractures, weight bearing is allowed at week 3.

INTRODUCTION

The ankle represents the most commonly injured weight-bearing joint in the human body. Ankle fracture treatment is still controversial, leading to severe arthritis when it is not properly addressed. Ankle fractures are typically the result of low-energy, rotational injury mechanisms. However, ankle fractures represent a spectrum of injury patterns from simple to very complex, with varying incidence of posttraumatic arthritis.[1] Stable injury patterns can be treated nonoperatively; unstable injury patterns are typically treated operatively. An epidemiologic study of 1500 ankle fractures revealed that isolated distal fibular or lateral malleolus fractures occurred in two-thirds of patients, whereas bimalleolar fractures occurred in a quarter and trimalleolar fractures in the remaining 7%.[2]

Disclosure: The authors have nothing to disclose.
Orthopaedic Department, Clínica Alemana de Santiago, Universidad del Desarrollo, Vitacura 5957, Santiago, Chile 7650568
* Corresponding author.
E-mail address: cortiz@alemana.cl

Foot Ankle Clin N Am 21 (2016) 367–389
http://dx.doi.org/10.1016/j.fcl.2016.01.008
1083-7515/16/$ – see front matter © 2016 Elsevier Inc. All rights reserved.

foot.theclinics.com

The epidemiologic situation in Chile and South America is similar to the rest of the world. However, not every patient has immediate access to a high level of quality medical care, because there is an obvious limit in the availability of resources, as well as a scarcity of well-trained foot and ankle or trauma surgeons. In South America, the use of expensive implants is generally restricted, but some private practice institutions have implants available from around the world, regardless of cost.

In this article, each fracture type is covered separately depending on its anatomic location (ie lateral malleolus, medial malleolus, posterior malleolus and syndesmosis), ending with a discussion of rehabilitation.

Lateral Malleolus Fracture

Introduction

Supination-external rotation (SER) injuries of the ankle comprise 40% to 55% of malleolar fractures.[3]

Approximately 85% of fractures of the lateral malleolus occur without substantial injury to the medial side of the ankle joint.[4,5] Several investigators have described that most ankle fractures follow the patterns described by Lauge-Hansen.[6] However, there are several fractures that do not exactly follow this classification. Despite this, Lauge-Hansen's[6] classification is useful to understand the mechanism of injury and how it progresses from a low-energy into a higher energy fracture; therefore, surgeons can anticipate both radiographic and anatomic changes in surgery.

Pathomechanics

The rationale for operating on ankle fractures is based on the classic study by Ramsey and Hamilton,[7] in which 1 mm of talar shift resulted in a 42% decrease in tibiotalar contact surface area, information that has been further confirmed recently.[8] In addition, there are several clinical studies suggesting that radiographic signs of ankle osteoarthritis occur when there are ankle malunions with greater than 1 or 2 mm of lateral talar shift.[9-12] Substantial lateral displacement of the talus can alter tibiotalar joint dynamics in isolated fibular fractures, even with an intact deltoid ligament (DL). This decrease in contact area gives an increase in force per unit area, generating high-stress concentrations on articular cartilage, which can lead to arthritis in the short or long term.[8,13] Based on this previous evidence, 1 mm of talar shift has become the recognized indication for operative fixation, which in turn was assumed to result from 1 to 2 mm of lateral fibular displacement in any radiograph view.

The 2-mm limit of fibular fracture displacement has been suggested by many investigators.[14,15] However, in 2010, van den Bekerom and van Dijk[16] showed that in Lauge-Hansen–type SER stage II with an intact DL more than 2 mm of fibular displacement can be observed without any displacement at the joint with an intact medial space (**Fig. 1**). Another study showed that displacement at the fibular fracture is caused by medialization and internal rotation of the proximal fragment and that the relation between the talus and the distal fibula remains intact.[15] Therefore, indications for the operative treatment of ankle fractures based solely on lateral malleolar displacement might not be reliable, because the stabilizing role of the DL has to be evaluated first.[16] This has been confirmed further in the literature, in which a surgically created fibular osteotomy with up to 6 mm of displacement did not cause a substantial change in tibiotalar contact area, but sectioning of the DL, regardless of fibular displacement, did create a decrease in contact area.[17] Considering this evidence, when there is a bimalleolar ankle fracture or its equivalent DL rupture, joint displacement is expected and surgery is an absolute indication, because complete medial instability will be observed.[16]

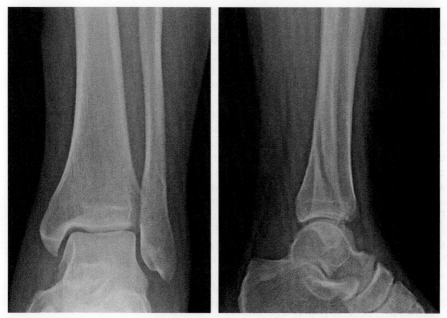

Fig. 1. Anteroposterior (AP) (*left*)/lateral (*right*) ankle radiograph showing nondisplaced lateral malleolar fracture.

Management

The senior authors recommend conservative treatment when there is a competent medial side with no joint incongruity, which represents a stable fracture (**Fig. 2**); unstable injury patterns are typically treated operatively. To determine whether an ankle fracture is unstable and surgery is indicated, clinical and radiographic analysis must be performed. Clinical conditions such as age, presence of osteoporosis, and diabetes should be considered in surgical planning. In clinical examination, functional compromise, such as inability to bear weight, suggests an unstable fracture.

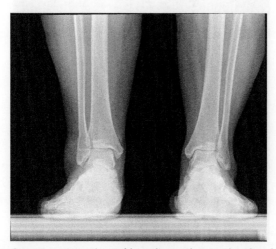

Fig. 2. Weight-bearing AP comparative ankle radiograph 6 weeks after fracture.

In radiographic evaluation, joint congruency must be evaluated independent of fibular displacement. Weight-bearing anteroposterior (AP), oblique, and lateral ankle radiographs are the standard films required. Several parameters have to be measured. These parameters include medial clear space, tibiofibular overlap and clear space, amount of fibular fracture displacement, and fibular length (using the talocrural angle). The width of the medial clear space, defined as the distance between the lateral border of the medial malleolus and the medial border of the talus at the level of the talar dome with the ankle in dorsiflexion, is considered to be representative of the status of the deep DL. An absolute width of the medial clear space more than 4 to 5 mm on weight-bearing or stress radiographs suggests deep DL rupture and the need for operative treatment[15,18] (**Fig. 3**). The authors believe that an increased medial clear space is not an absolute indication for surgery. Instead, the authors perform surgery when there is an increased medial clear space compared with the contralateral side or an asymmetric joint comparing its medial, lateral, and superior joint spaces. Regarding the tibiofibular overlap (>1 mm on oblique radiographs and >5 mm on AP radiographs) and tibiofibular clear space (<5 mm on AP radiographs), it is important to compare these with the contralateral side given that some normal patients do not have tibiofibular overlap. Regarding fibular length, there is some information available[19,20] that a shortened fibula (>5 mm) can end in a valgus ankle. Fibular length is measured by the talocrural angle, the angle formed between an intermalleolar line (from medial malleolus to lateral malleolus tip) and a distal tibia joint line. The normal range for these values is 8° to 15°.

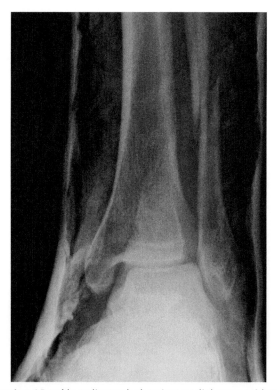

Fig. 3. Weight-bearing AP ankle radiograph showing medial space widening.

In the absence of distinct radiographic widening of the medial space and asymmetry of the ankle mortise, gravity stress radiographs can be beneficial if there is any doubt about ankle stability (**Fig. 4**).[15] Other investigators have advocated external rotation stress radiographs. More recent studies have suggested that the gravity stress test is as reliable as the external rotation stress test, more comfortable for the patient, and easy to perform by radiograph technicians. This test is simple, reproducible, and does not require the surgeon to be present to perform the test. It is our preference to make the final confirmation of an unstable ankle with minimal fibular fracture displacement.[21–23] Intraoperatively, external rotation views are easy to obtain. It is important to perform this external rotation with ankle dorsiflexion and hindfoot varus.[24,25]

In the absence of an open injury or irreducible dislocation, surgical treatment of an unstable ankle fracture pattern is not an emergency and can be completed as a scheduled outpatient procedure. The authors choose to perform surgery when the soft tissues allow a positive wrinkle test.

The current standard in treating unstable fractures is through open reduction and internal fixation (ORIF) with plates and screws. The principles for lateral malleolus fractures classically follow the arbeitsgemeinschaft fur osteosynthesefragen (AO) principles that include atraumatic soft tissue handling with minimal periosteal stripping, anatomic fracture reduction, sufficiently rigid internal fixation, and early range of motion.[26]

Restoration of fibular length and rotation is critical in reestablishing a stable ankle mortise, and can be assessed radiographically. In the presence of severe comminution, the authors use traction and indirect reduction, using the other ankle as a reference. If possible, fixation begins with an interfragmentary fixation screw to allow compression at the fracture site. Fibular stabilization can be completed using either a posterior antiglide or lateral neutralization technique, typically with a simple one-third tubular plate and 3.5-mm cortical screws (**Fig. 5**).

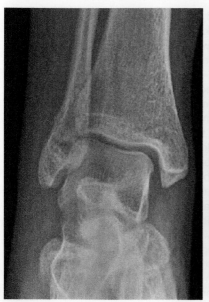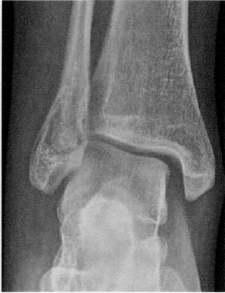

Fig. 4. (*Left*) Normal-looking AP ankle radiograph showing no medial space widening. (*Right*) Gravity stress radiograph: in the same ankle, when positioned on lateral decubitus and left unsupported, a medial space opening can be seen.

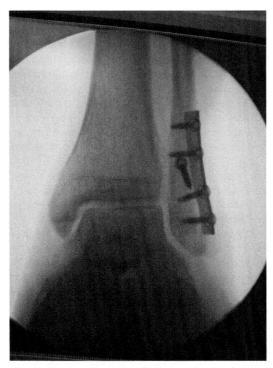

Fig. 5. AP ankle radiograph showing classic lateral malleolus fixation, with a one-third tubular plate and an interfragmentary screw.

In 2014, Huang and colleagues[27] compared 3 different plates for fibular fractures in 147 patients, showing better results using locking compression plates compared with nonlocking tubular plates. Even better results were obtained with the locking anatomic fibular plate. This plate is particularly useful in osteoporotic bones, multiple fracture fragments, or for small distal fragments.[27]

Although posterior plating has been indicated to increase construct stability, the authors think that there is a higher risk of peroneal irritation. The authors prefer to increase construct stability by using an anatomic locking plate when needed (**Fig. 6**). The cost of the implant must be considered because it is considerably higher than that of the typical one-third tubular plate. Most investigators begin with fixation of the lateral malleolus. Clinicians could consider starting with fixation of the medial or posterior malleolus if severe comminution or bone loss of the lateral malleolus is present. Even though some investigators have advocated fixation for high fibular fractures,[1] the authors think the risk of peroneal nerve injury is too great to perform fixation of fractures at the midportion of the fibula.

Occasionally, the fibula in a Weber B or a low Weber C fracture can be approached with a percutaneous or minimally invasive approach. Using fluoroscopic control, the fibular fracture is percutaneously reduced with a reduction forceps. The distal fragment needs to be manipulated to gain length and internally rotated. If successful, a percutaneous lag screw is placed from anterior to posterior, perpendicular to the fracture, then a percutaneous plate should be used.[28] Intramedullary fixation of distal fibular fractures has been shown to have outcomes similar to modern plating techniques. However, there is unconvincing evidence that percutaneous intramedullary

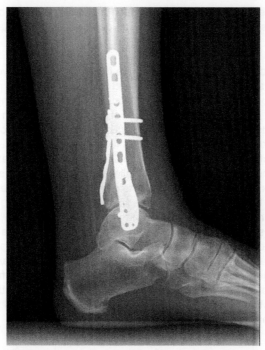

Fig. 6. Lateral ankle radiograph showing an anatomic locked distal fibular plate on an elderly patient. The posterior tibial plate is described elsewhere.

fixation is superior to standard techniques with regard to clinical and functional outcome. The authors think that it should be considered as one of the minimally invasive options to use when there is severe soft tissue damage.[29]

Ankle fractures in diabetics is an extensive topic, so only general recommendations from the Wukich and Kline[30] article are discussed here. Diabetic patients without neuropathy and/or vasculopathy have a similar outcome to nondiabetic patients. If vasculopathy and/or neuropathy are present, a higher postoperative complication risk exists (25%–40%), including a 5% risk of amputation. Complications can be divided into those related to soft tissue or bone. Bone complications include, but are not limited to, Charcot arthropathy, malunions, nonunions or delayed unions (30%), arthrodesis, and osteomyelitis. Soft tissue complications include infections (15%–30%) and wound dehiscence. For surgical treatment, supplemental fixation is used to avoid bone complications. This supplementation consists of multiple syndesmotic screws, transarticular fixation, supplemental external fixation devices, and locked plates. Postoperatively, a non–weight-bearing period of at least 6 to 12 weeks followed by protected weight bearing is prudent.

Medial Malleolus Fracture/Deltoid Ligament Rupture

Introduction
The medial ankle complex consists of the medial malleolus (MM) and the DL. The medial ankle column is an integral part of the ankle mortise. The DL is a ligament complex that consists of 2 layers: superficial and deep. The superficial layer consists of the tibionavicular, tibiospring, tibiocalcaneal, and the superficial posterior tibiotalar

ligament. The deep layer consists of the deep anterior and posterior tibiotalar ligaments. The largest band of the DL is the deep posterior tibiotalar ligament.

Pathomechanics

Rasmussen and colleagues[31] investigated the function of the DL layers.[31,32] The superficial DL resists eversion of the hindfoot and the deep layer is the primary restraint to external rotation of the talus.[33] Close[34] found that, after sectioning all lateral ligaments, an intact deltoid allows only 2 mm of separation between talus and MM. When the deep deltoid is sectioned, the talus separates 3.7 mm from the MM. The DL also participates in the coupling between foot and tibia. If the DL is cut, the foot-tibia motion significantly changes during dorsiflexion and plantarflexion.[35] The MM comprises the tension side and the lateral malleolus the compression side of the ankle. There is no compression and no weight transfer through the MM. There are only traction forces going through it. Regarding the MM-DL relation, the bigger the MM fracture, the less ligamentous lesion exists, and vice versa. That is why, with very small collicular fractures, a DL incompetence has to be ruled out before a pure fracture is diagnosed. Isolated medial malleolar fractures or DLs ruptures are rare. They usually occur as part of a bimalleolar or trimalleolar ankle fracture. They can be the consequence of a Lauge-Hansen adduction-supination type (vertical MM fracture pattern), a SER type 4, a pronation-abduction, and a pronation–external rotation type of fracture (transverse MM fracture). In all these types of fractures, an MM fracture or a DL rupture (medial malleolar equivalent) can happen.

Management

The diagnostic studies are the same for all ankle fractures and are discussed earlier. As shown by DeAngelis and colleagues,[36] medial tenderness has no value in identifying unstable DL rupture.[36] As stated earlier, the MM is the tension side of the ankle. No weight is transferred through this part of the joint. For this reason, isolated MM displacements under the joint shoulder do not necessarily need to be fixed. It is not a weight-bearing surface, and, with the broad DL insertion on the MM, a stable ankle is in most cases observed. If in doubt, stress views can be obtained. Isolated displaced MM fractures at or above the medial corner of the ankle joint should be fixed given its weight-bearing surface and the consequent medial ankle incompetence.

In cases of unimalleolar lateral malleolar fractures with a congruent joint (no increased medial clear space) and a lateral malleolar displacement (>2 mm), DL status has to be investigated. This investigation can be done with stress views, as stated earlier. If an instability is shown, the lateral malleolus has to be fixed and the syndesmosis should be stressed to uncover any instability. If a stable syndesmosis is shown, no further treatment is necessary. The authors do not repair the DL if a stable syndesmosis is evident with a congruent joint. We allow the DL to heal without any surgical intervention. Stromsoe and colleagues[37] showed, in a randomized study of 50 patients, that no difference exists repairing the DL. They concluded that operative repair of the deltoid was unnecessary as long as the mortise anatomy was reestablished. Nevertheless, the investigators recognized that there is a small group of patients (to be determined) who persist with medial gutter pain or medial instability. In bimalleolar and trimalleolar fractures there is little discussion about the surgical decision if a displaced MM is found, because this indicates ankle instability. In cases of undisplaced or minimally displaced MM fractures under the shoulder joint, nonoperative treatment is a valid option.[38]

Regarding technical details, a myriad of surgical options exist, including isolated Kirschner wires (K-wires); K-wires with screws; tension band technique; headless, partially threaded, or fully threaded screws; cannulated or solid screws; low-profile plates; claw plates; cerclage techniques. Studies have shown that neutralization plates are more stable than screws.[39–41] The tension band technique is useful in small MM fragments. FiberWire or K-wires can be used for tensioning; however, K-wires were shown to be a more rigid construct than FiberWire.[42] Screws are the most frequently used surgical solutions for MM fractures (**Fig. 7**). Normally, partially threaded screws are enough and easy to use. Biomechanical studies found that bicortical screws are more stable than unicortical partially threaded screws, but no clinical difference has been shown with this technique.[42,43] Headless compression screws provide good clinical results, but no clinical difference has been shown with this technique if headed screws are buried under the DL and sunk into the bone intraoperatively.[44] The screw position is important but not crucial for the MM reduction. Divergent screws are more stable than parallel or convergent screws in a biomechanical study.[45]

The surgical approach normally used is a straight medial incision. If screws are used, a 2-cm longitudinal incision is generally enough to allow an adequate ankle joint exposure (joint shoulder) and fracture visualization to achieve a perfect fracture reduction. If a plate is used, a 3-cm to 4-cm incision length will be necessary. A valid option is to use a minimally invasive anteromedial approach (5 mm) to visualize just the joint shoulder. This approach aids with the joint and fracture reduction.[46]

Ankle arthroscopy can help to make diagnoses such as medial ankle instability and chondral lesions. It is also useful to aid with anatomic fracture reduction and percutaneous fixation.[28,47] Contraindications for arthroscopic assistance are a grossly compromised soft tissue envelope and a fracture that is significantly displaced that evidently indicates ORIF. Clinicians must be aware of the necessity of greater radiological exposure and the risk of technical errors with inexperienced surgeons, compared with ORIF.[48]

Posterior Malleolar Fractures

Introduction
Posterior malleolar fractures have been increasingly considered in ankle fracture management in the last 5 years, because of increased understanding of the factors

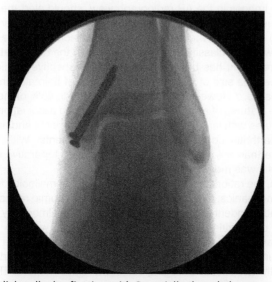

Fig. 7. Classic medial malleolus fixation with 2 partially threaded screws.

governing ankle stability and biomechanics. There is a lack of evidence for when and how to treat this component of ankle fractures. Isolated posterior malleolar fractures have been described in parachute landings because of the energy involved, in up to 41% of ankle fractures.[49] The frequency of posterior malleolar involvement in ankle fractures can be up to 50% as reported recently.[50]

Pathomechanics

A better understanding of the anatomy of the posterior ankle joint has been paramount in understanding the pathomechanics of posterior ankle fractures. Some of the knowledge in this area of the ankle has been highlighted by hindfoot arthroscopy articles such as the ones by van Dijk,[51] in which the importance of the ligaments that make up a labrum for the posterior ankle has been stressed. The most frequently injured part of the posterior ankle malleolus is the posterolateral fragment, where the posteroinferior tibiofibular ligament is inserted. In rotationally unstable ankle fractures without posterior malleolus fractures, the posteroinferior tibiofibular ligament (PITFL) is damaged as a delamination off the posterior malleolus, which understates the importance of this ligament in providing stability for the ankle.[52] When the fragment containing the PITFL is reduced and fixed, the stability of the ankle is greatly improved[53] and it has already been shown that the PITFL alone makes up 42% of the strength of the syndesmosis.[54] When syndesmotic stability in ankle fractures is clinically evaluated, posterior malleolar fixation is at least equivalent to syndesmotic screw stabilization. Avoiding a syndesmotic screw avoids the need for subsequent screw removal or inadequate reduction.[55] Regarding cartilage damage and arthritic changes, the instability created after a posterior malleolar fracture may be more important than the step-off at the fracture site. This possibility has been suggested by the observation that medial and lateral constraints are more important in preventing posterior talus translation after posterior malleolar fractures than the articular surface compromise.[56]

Management

Incongruences of the posterior aspect of the pilon on the lateral radiograph view, or linear radiodense images in the AP radiograph view, should alert the surgeon to the presence of posterior column damage (**Fig. 8**). It is our practice to perform computed tomography (CT) scans whenever a posterior malleolus fracture is suspected, because this allows us to classify and better decide on the best treatment.

Conservative treatment has been evaluated in retrospective studies, showing no correlation between the size of the gap or percentage of tibiotalar area compromise and the clinical results.[57] However, in this same study up to 63% of the cases showed some radiological features of arthritis. In a recent study, an association was found between ankle fractures with larger posterior malleolus fragments and an increased frequency of osteoarthritis compared with smaller fragments. With fragment sizes representing more than 5% of the tibiotalar area and postoperative step-off greater than 1 mm, arthritis was more frequent.[58]

For the authors, the rationale for treating posterior ankle malleolus fractures should be based on biomechanics. Our objective is to obtain anatomic reduction of the posterior malleolus independent of the fragment size, because almost any fracture size increases the risk of arthritis. Haraguchi and colleagues[59] was the first to classify posterior malleolar fractures of the ankle into posterolateral-oblique (type 1), transverse medial-extension (type 2), and small-shell (type 3) fractures. Bartoníček and colleagues[60] recently proposed a slightly different classification. The analysis by Mangnus and colleagues[61] brings more clarity to the analysis, stating that because

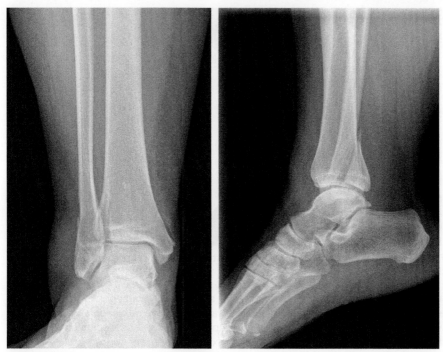

Fig. 8. AP ankle radiograph (*left*) showing a linear radiodensity on the distal tibia, indicating a hidden posterior malleolus fracture. Lateral ankle radiograph (*right*) showing a posterior malleolus fracture.

of the intrinsic instability generated by a transverse fracture exiting through the MM, separating the anterior from the posterior colliculus and therefore compromising the insertion of the deep deltoid, these fractures should be considered for fixation (**Fig. 9**). In contrast, fractures not compromising the MM could be evaluated for their medial stability and therefore surgery could be deemed unnecessary in some cases.

Regarding surgical technique, for posterolateral fragments, Haraguchi type 1, the authors commonly perform surgical reduction through the lateral approach commonly performed for the lateral malleolus. We perform a slightly posterolateral incision over the fibula in order to have access both to the posterior part of the fibula and the posterior tibial fragment, and therefore are able to achieve reduction of the posterior tibial fragment with clamps or pointed instruments. Another surgical option for small posterolateral fragments is to perform an indirect reduction and a minimally invasive fixation when the fragments are amenable to fixation (ie, the fragment measures more than 10–15 mm in any direction). In these cases, anterior-to-posterior or posterior-to-anterior percutaneous screws are used.

For posterior central or posterior medial fragments, the authors prefer a separate approach from the classic medial or lateral approaches; either a posterolateral or posteromedial exposure. When the fracture mainly compromises the MM, behaving like a sagittal split, and there is a marginal posterior component, the classic medial approach for the MM suffices and the MM is fixed with mini fragment screws, 2.4 mm or 2.7 mm, in an anterior-to-posterior direction besides the classic interfragmentary oblique distal-to-proximal screws. When the posterior component is amenable to fixation and

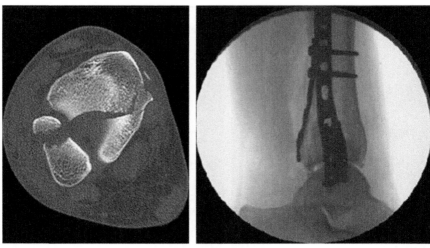

Fig. 9. (*Left*) CT scan of a Haraguchi type 2 posterior malleolus fracture. (*Right*) After fixation with a one-third tubular buttress plate.

mainly posteromedial in location, the senior authors prefer a separate posteromedial approach (just posterior to the tibialis posterior) to achieve reduction and stabilization with a small fragment plate. This plate is supposed to work as a buttress plate, and, therefore, after reduction of the fragment, proximal fixation is enough to achieve pretensioning of the plate in order to hold the posterior malleolus fragment in place (see **Fig. 9**).[62] If the posterior component is amenable to fixation and essentially posterior in location, the authors prefer a classic posterolateral approach, which is our preferred exposure. In the authors' opinion, performing a posterolateral approach to reduce and fix both the fibula and the posterior malleolus is technically difficult and, when fixing the 3 malleoli, the authors prefer a straight posterolateral approach for the posterior fragment, a straight lateral approach for the fibular fracture, and a medial incision for the MM (**Fig. 10**). The fracture fixation order should be to first start with fibular interfragmentary screws, followed by the posterior malleolus fixation, and then the lateral fibular plate. This order is followed to avoid radiograph obstruction of the posterior malleolar fracture reduction by the lateral fibular plate.

The authors indicate arthroscopically assisted fixation of posterior malleolar fractures when there is minimal displacement and when the complete fracture treatment is amenable to minimally invasive treatment.

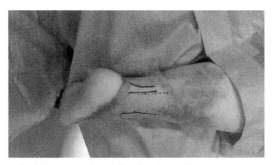

Fig. 10. Posterolateral approach as shown by the dotted line, lateral to the Achilles tendon. This approach is separate to the direct lateral approach.

Syndesmotic Injury

Introduction

Syndesmotic injury is a complex subtopic of ankle fractures, requiring understanding of its anatomy, injury mechanism, reduction maneuvers, stabilization methods, and hardware removal timing.

Starting with the syndesmosis anatomy, it comprises the distal aspect of the fibula and the concave lateral aspect of the distal tibia. Widening of the syndesmosis by 1 mm decreases the joint contact area by 42%, with a probable secondary overload and instability and hence early osteoarthritis of the tibiotalar joint.[7,8,13] The syndesmosis comprises 4 ligaments: interosseous, anterior-inferior, posteroinferior, and transverse ligaments. The anterior-inferior and posteroinferior ligaments contribute 35% and 33% to ankle stability respectively.[54,63,64]

Pathomechanics

The most common injury mechanism is external rotation and dorsiflexion. These mechanisms can end in fractures or sprains (so called high ankle sprains). A thorough physical examination and radiograph analysis has to be performed for proper diagnosis. The most common physical assessments are the external rotation stress and the squeeze tests. The first test comprises external rotation of the foot with the knee in 90° of flexion,[65] and the latter test entails a tibia and fibula proximal compression, looking for ankle syndesmosis referred pain in both tests. Nevertheless, even 20% of syndesmotic injuries are overlooked if only physical examination and no radiograph is performed.[66] Radiographic parameters are discussed earlier in this article.[67,68] The most reliable measurement is the tibiofibular clear space.[69] When there is any doubt on syndesmotic stability, a comparative CT scan is performed. CT scan can detect minimal diastasis.[70] Intraoperative syndesmotic evaluation must always be performed. The most common examinations are the hook test and the external rotation test, both with poor sensitivity.[71] The authors use a more controlled test for syndesmotic evaluation. It is performed by introducing a soft tissue retractor (eg, a Farabeuf or Hohman retractor) into the syndesmosis and rotating it slowly under fluoroscopy (**Fig. 11**). Given its more controlled motion, this test allows much easier visualization of the syndesmosis stability. Some evidence also suggests that sagittal

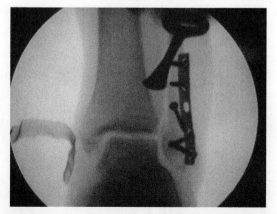

Fig. 11. Cotton test performed on fluoroscopy. A Hohman, Farabeuf, or Cobb instrument is inserted in the syndesmosis. By rotating it, a tibiofibular stress is applied in a controlled fashion.

plane instability must also be assessed by evaluating the AP motion of the fibula on the lateral radiograph.[72]

Management

Surgical treatment is performed on any unstable syndesmosis. It has been shown that an adequate syndesmotic reduction is correlated with better functional outcomes, less arthritis, and long-term stability of the syndesmosis.[73,74] Syndesmotic malreduction was shown to be associated with poor outcomes.[75,76] This phenomenon is probably caused by a significant increase in the mean contact pressures combined with a shift in the center of pressure of the fibula and talus.[77]

Regarding syndesmotic reduction, a cadaveric study found that a clamp compressing the fibula against the tibia, placed at 15° and 30° of angulation in the axial plane, generates malreductions in external rotation, however small in magnitude.[78] Placing the clamp in neutral generates the most accurate reduction.[79] Even with a good fluoroscopic result, the syndesmosis can be malreduced. A retrospective study showed that 33% of patients with ankle fractures with syndesmotic damage after adequate fluoroscopic reduction ended up with a syndesmotic malreduction.[80] The ways to improve reduction are direct visualization, contralateral comparison, intraoperative three-dimensional imaging, and intraoperative CT scans (**Fig. 12**).[81–83] Sagi and colleagues[74] found that, at 2 years' follow-up, patients with malreduced syndesmosis had worse functional results. The gold standard fixation method is syndesmotic screws. These screws are placed through the syndesmosis from the fibula to the tibia. They can vary in composition (metal or bioabsorbable materials), number (1 or 2 screws), size (3.5 or 4.5 mm diameter), location (trans-syndesmotic or suprasyndesmotic), and type (lag screw or situation screw), and may be tricortical or quatricortical screws. No major differences exist in functional outcomes between these different types of fixation.[84–95] Only Schepers and colleagues[96] found that screw placement 41 mm above the syndesmosis negatively influenced outcome. The investigators recommended positioning the syndesmotic screw 2 cm proximal to the ankle joint. A stronger fixation is achieved with lag screws, 4.5-mm screws, and double screws. Two-hole or 3-hole plates with screws are more stable than 4.5-mm screws alone[97,98] (**Fig. 13**). The investigators think that only in certain cases, as in obesity or Charcot arthropathy, are these strong fixation options necessary.[99,100] Suture buttons allow reliable and strong fixation,[101] starting posteriorly on the fibula and ending anteromedial on the tibia (**Fig. 14**).[102] Long-term results show similar functional scores

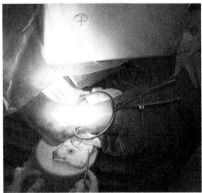
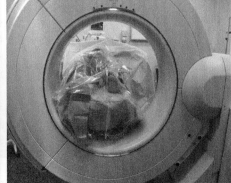

Fig. 12. Intraoperative view of syndesmotic clamp in place (*Left*) and CT scan (*Right*).

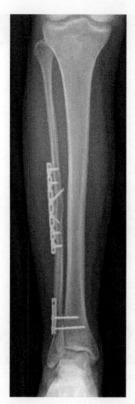

Fig. 13. Two syndesmotic screws through a 3-hole one-third tubular plate.

comparing suture button and screws, with a lower removal rate. Some studies show that patients return to work more quickly and experience better clinical outcomes.[63,103–106] Peterson showed that there is some increase in tibiofibular clear space relative to the initial postfixation position, but with no consequence for the short-term follow-up (3 years).[106]

The high rate of postoperative syndesmosis malreduction has already been discussed, even under adequate fluoroscopy. The standard method to diagnose a malreduction on CT scan remains a matter of debate and none is universally accepted.[107,108] An easy and reproducible parameter is to draw a line that follows the anterolateral border of the fibula. If this line is within 2 mm of the anterolateral border of the tibia, it is considered normal. More than 2 mm was abnormal in 100% of cases.[109]

Hardware failure and screw removal are also controversial topics. Screw breakage occurs in around 20% of cases. There is no difference in functional advantage between patients with screws removed and retained, but other studies have shown that patients with broken screws have better functional scores that the ones with retained screws.[110–112] Removing screws is probably beneficial for syndesmosis motion and to correct malreduction induced by screw fixation.[113] Song and colleagues[113] showed that screw removal allows syndesmosis reduction in 90% of malreduced syndesmoses, but there is no evident benefit comparing screw removal with broken screws. In patients with intact screws that cause irritation, it is probably prudent to remove them,[114,115] although a 22% complication rate is associated with this

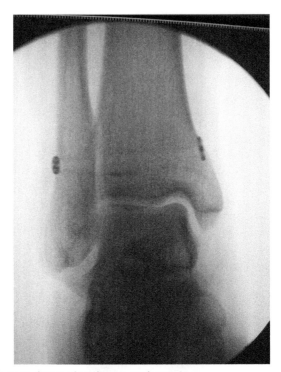

Fig. 14. Suture button device placed on a syndesmosis.

procedure (9% infection rate).[116] In contrast, if screws are removed beforehand (before 12 weeks) a recurrent diastasis can occur. Screw removal at 6 weeks reduces the rate of implant failure but increases the rate of diastasis.[117,118] The authors only remove syndesmotic screws if they become symptomatic, or if they become loose or break at 6 months after surgery.

Postoperative Management/Rehabilitation

As shown by Pfeifer and colleagues[119] and Lin and colleages,[120] there is no consensus in the literature regarding rehabilitation protocols. Just a few articles report accelerated functional rehabilitation.[121] The classic recommendation is non–weight bearing in a cast or brace for 6 weeks.[122] The DL and the posterior syndesmosis play key roles in the stability of ankle fractures. If these structures remain intact, early functional treatment is completely safe. It has been shown that full weight bearing is not associated with increased morbidity or loss of reduction. Furthermore, patients with early weight bearing and ankle motion have better ankle dorsiflexion at 12 weeks and quicker return to work compared with cast immobilization cases.[123] However, early motion is associated with an increased risk of wound infection/dehiscence.[124]

The authors adhere to an accelerated rehabilitation protocol. For stable (nonsurgical) and operatively treated unimalleolar fractures, weight bearing as tolerated is allowed as soon as possible (first postoperative day). A walker boot is used as immobilization for 3 weeks. Range of motion is allowed immediately for nonoperative fractures, and delayed for 2 weeks in surgically treated unimalleolar fractures until wound healing is observed.

For bimalleolar or trimalleolar fractures, as well as fixed syndesmosis, weight bearing is delayed for 3 weeks in a walking boot. Weight bearing in simulated models has shown that the posterior one-fourth of the ankle joint remains unloaded with axial load. This finding supports the idea that weight bearing, even in surgically repaired posterior malleolar fractures, is not harmful.[125] The walker boot is used from weeks 3 to 6. After this period, an ankle brace is suggested for 1 more month. Physical therapy is suggested starting at week 3.

REFERENCES

1. Clare MP. A rational approach to ankle fractures. Foot Ankle Clin 2008;13(4): 593–610.
2. Court-Brown CM, McBirnie J, Wilson G. Adult ankle fractures–an increasing problem? Acta Orthop Scand 1998;69(1):43–7.
3. Moody ML, Koeneman J, Hettinger E, et al. The effects of fibular and talar displacement on joint contact areas about the ankle. Orthop Rev 1992;21: 741–4.
4. Michelson JD, Helgemo SL. Kinematics of the axially loaded ankle. Foot Ankle Int 1995;16(9):577–82.
5. Harper MC. The short oblique fracture of the distal fibula without medial injury: an assessment of displacement. Foot Ankle Int 1995;16(4):181–6.
6. Lauge-Hansen N. Fractures of the ankle II: combined experimental-surgical and experimental-roentgenologic investigations. Arch Surg 1950;60(5):957–85.
7. Ramsey PL, Hamilton W. Changes in tibiotalar area of contact caused by lateral talar shift. J Bone Joint Surg Am 1976;58(3):356–7.
8. Lloyd J, Elsayed S, Hariharan K, et al. Revisiting the concept of talar shift in ankle fractures. Foot Ankle Int 2006;27(10):793–6.
9. Hughes JL, Weber H, Willenegger H, et al. Evaluation of ankle fractures: non-operative and operative treatment. Clin Orthop Relat Res 1979;(138):111–9.
10. Joy G, Patzakis MJ, Harvey JP Jr. Precise evaluation of the reduction of severe ankle fractures. Technique and correlation with end results. J Bone Joint Surg Am 1974;56(5):979–93.
11. Pettrone FA, Gail M, Pee D, et al. Quantitative criteria for prediction of the results after displaced fracture of the ankle. J Bone Joint Surg Am 1983;65(5):667–77.
12. Wilson FC Jr, Skilbred LA. Long-term results in the treatment of displaced bimalleolar fractures. J Bone Joint Surg Am 1966;48(6):1065–78.
13. Harris J, Fallat L. Effects of isolated Weber B fibular fractures on the tibiotalar contact area. J Foot Ankle Surg 2004;43(1):3–9.
14. Thordason DB, Motamed S, Hedman T, et al. The effect of fibular malreduction on contact pressures in an ankle fracture malunion model. J Bone Joint Surg Am 1997;79(12):1809–15.
15. Michelson JD, Varner KE, Checcone M. Diagnosing deltoid injury in ankle fractures: the gravity stress view. Clin Orthop Relat Res 2001;(387):178–82.
16. van den Bekerom MP, van Dijk CN. Is fibular fracture displacement consistent with tibiotalar displacement? Clin Orthop Relat Res 2010;468(4):969–74.
17. Clarke HJ, Michelson JD, Cox QG, et al. Tibio-talar stability in bimalleolar ankle fractures: a dynamic in vitro contact area study. Foot Ankle 1991;11(4):222–7.
18. Egol KA, Amirtharajah M, Tejwani NC, et al. Ankle stress test for predicting the need for surgical fixation of isolated fibular fractures. J Bone Joint Surg Am 2004;86-A(11):2393–8.

19. Dias LS. Valgus deformity of the ankle joint: pathogenesis of fibular shortening. J Pediatr Orthop 1985;5(2):176–80.

20. Park HW, Kim HW, Kwak YH, et al. Ankle valgus deformity secondary to proximal migration of the fibula in tibial lengthening with use of the Ilizarov external fixator. J Bone Joint Surg Am 2011;93(3):294–302.

21. Gill JB, Risko T, Raducan V, et al. Comparison of manual and gravity stress radiographs for the evaluation of supination-external rotation fibular fractures. J Bone Joint Surg Am 2007;89(5):994–9.

22. Schock HJ, Pinzur M, Manion L, et al. The use of gravity or manual-stress radiographs in the assessment of supination-external rotation fractures of the ankle. J Bone Joint Surg Br 2007;89(8):1055–9.

23. Koval KJ, Egol KA, Cheung Y, et al. Does a positive ankle stress test indicate the need for operative treatment after lateral malleolus fracture? A preliminary report. J Orthop Trauma 2007;21(7):449–55.

24. Park SS, Kubiak EN, Egol KA, et al. Stress radiographs after ankle fracture: the effect of ankle position and deltoid ligament status on medial clear space measurements. J Orthop Trauma 2006;20(1):11–8.

25. Femino JE, Vaseenon T, Phisitkul P, et al. Varus external rotation stress test for radiographic detection of deep deltoid ligament disruption with and without syndesmotic disruption: a cadaveric study. Foot Ankle Int 2013;34(2):251–60.

26. Perren SM. Basic aspects of internal fixation. In: Müller ME, Allgower M, Schneider R, et al, editors. Manual of internal fixation. 3rd edition. New York: Springer-Verlag; 1991. p. 1–112.

27. Huang ZeYu, Liu Lei, Tu ChongQi, et al. Comparison of three plate system for lateral malleolar fixation. BMC Musculoskelet Disord 2014;15:360.

28. Gumann G, Hamilton GA. Arthroscopically assisted treatment of ankle injuries. Clin Podiatr Med Surg 2011;28(3):523–38.

29. Jain S, Haughton BA, Brew C. Intramedullary fixation of distal fibular fractures: a systematic review of clinical and functional outcomes. J Orthop Traumatol 2014; 15(4):245–54.

30. Wukich DK, Kline AJ. The management of ankle fractures in patients with diabetes. J Bone Joint Surg Am 2008;90(7):1570–8.

31. Rasmussen O, Kroman-Andersen C, Boe S. Deltoid ligament: functional analysis of the medial collateral ligamentous apparatus of the ankle joint. Acta Orthop Scand 1983;54:36.

32. Rasmussen O. Stability of the ankle joint: analysis of the function and traumatology of the ankle ligaments. Acta Orthop Scand 1985;56(Suppl 2):1–75.

33. Hintermann B. Medial ankle instability. Foot Ankle Clin 2003;8(4):723–38.

34. Close JR. Some applications of the functional anatomy of the ankle joint. J Bone Joint Surg Am 1956;38A:761–81.

35. Hintermann B, Sommer C, Nigg BM. The influence of ligament transection on tibial and calcaneal rotation with loading and dorsi-plantarflexion. Foot Ankle 1995;16(7):567–71.

36. DeAngelis NA, Eskander MS, French BG. Does medial tenderness predict deep deltoid ligament incompetence in supination-external rotation type ankle fractures? J Orthop Trauma 2007;21(4):244–7.

37. Stromsoe K, Hoqevold HE, Skjeldal S, et al. The repair of a ruptured deltoid ligament is not necessary in ankle fractures. J Bone Joint Surg Br 1995;77(6): 920–1.

38. Hoelsbrekken SE, Kaul-Jensen K, Mørch T, et al. Nonoperative treatment of the medial malleolus in bimalleolar and trimalleolar ankle fractures: a randomized controlled trial. J Orthop Trauma 2013;27(11):633–7.

39. Dumigan RM, Bronson DG, Early JS. Analysis of fixation methods for vertical shear fractures of the medial malleolus. J Orthop Trauma 2006;20(10):687–91.

40. Georgiadis GM, White DB. Modified tension band wiring of medial malleolar ankle fractures. Foot Ankle Int 1995;16(2):64–8.

41. Patel T, Owen JR, Byrd WA, et al. Biomechanical performance of a new device for medial malleolar fractures. Foot Ankle Int 2013;34(3):426–33.

42. Fowler TT, Pugh KJ, Litsky AS, et al. Medial malleolar fractures: a biomechanical study of fixation techniques. Orthopedics 2011;34(8):e349–55.

43. Ricci WM, Tornetta P, Borrelli J Jr. Lag screw fixation of medial malleolar fractures: a biomechanical, radiographic, and clinical comparison of unicortical partially threaded lag screws and bicortical fully threaded lag screws. J Orthop Trauma 2012;26(10):602–6.

44. Barnes H, Cannada LK, Watson JT. A clinical evaluation of alternative fixation techniques for medial malleolus fractures. Injury 2014;45(9):1365–7.

45. Amanatullah DF, Khan SN, Curtiss S, et al. Effect of divergent screw fixation in vertical medial malleolus fractures. J Trauma Acute Care Surg 2012;72(3): 751–4.

46. Saini P, Aggrawal A, Meena S, et al. Miniarthrotomy assisted percutaneous screw fixation for displaced medial malleolus fractures - a novel technique. J Clin Orthop Trauma 2014;5(4):252–6.

47. Swart EF, Vosseller JT. Arthroscopic assessment of medial malleolar reduction. Arch Orthop Trauma Surg 2014;134(9):1287–92.

48. Szczęsny G, Janowicz J. Minimally invasive osteosynthesis of ankle fractures. Pol Orthop Traumatol 2012;77:145–50.

49. Young K, Kim J, Cho J, et al. Paratrooper's ankle fracture: posterior malleolar fracture. Clin Orthop Surg 2015;7:15–21.

50. Switaj PJ, Weatherford B, Fuchs D, et al. Evaluation of posterior malleolar fractures and the posterior pilon variant in operatively treated ankle fractures. Foot Ankle Int 2014;35(9):886–95.

51. van Dijk CN. Hindfoot endoscopy. Foot Ankle Clin North Am 2006;11:391–414.

52. Schottel P, Hinds R, Loftus M, et al. Analysis of PITFL injuries in rotationally unstable ankle fractures. Foot Ankle Int 2015;36(4):377–82.

53. Forberger J, Sabandal P, Dietrich M, et al. Posterolateral approach to the displaced posterior malleolus: functional outcome and local morbidity. Foot Ankle Int 2009;30(4):309–14.

54. Ogilvie-Harris DJ, Reed SC, Hedman TP. Disruption of the ankle syndesmosis: biomechanical study of the ligamentous restraints. Arthroscopy 1994;10(5): 558–60.

55. Miller AN, Carroll EA, Parker RJ, et al. Posterior malleolar stabilization of syndesmotic injuries is equivalent to screw fixation. Clin Orthop Relat Res 2010;468(4): 1129–35.

56. van den Bekerom MP, Haverkamp D, Kloen P. Biomechanical and clinical evaluation of posterior malleolar fractures. A systematic review of the literature. J Trauma 2009;66(1):279–84.

57. Donken CC, Goorden AJ, Verhofstad MH, et al. The outcome at 20 years of conservatively treated 'isolated' posterior malleolar fractures of the ankle. A case series. J Bone Joint Surg Br 2011;93(12):1621–5.

58. Drijfhout van Hooff CC, Verhage SM, Hoogendoorn JM. Influence of fragment size and postoperative joint congruency on long-term outcome of posterior malleolar fractures. Foot Ankle Int 2015;36(6):673–8.

59. Haraguchi N, Haruyama H, Toga H, et al. Pathoanatomy of posterior malleolar fractures of the ankle. J Bone Joint Surg Am 2006;88(5):1085–92.

60. Bartoníček J, Rammelt S, Kostlivý K, et al. Anatomy and classification of the posterior tibial fragment in ankle fractures. Arch Orthop Trauma Surg 2015;135(4):505–16.

61. Mangnus L, Meijer DT, Stufkens SA, et al. Posterior malleolar fracture patterns. J Orthop Trauma 2015;29(9):428–35.

62. Erdem MN, Erken HY, Burc H, et al. Comparison of lag screw versus buttress plate fixation of posterior malleolar fractures. Foot Ankle Int 2014;35(10):1022–30.

63. Van Heest TJ, Lafferty PM. Injuries to the ankle syndesmosis. J Bone Joint Surg Am 2014;96(7):603–13.

64. Hermans JJ, Beumer A, de Jong TA, et al. Anatomy of the distal tibiofibular syndesmosis in adults: a pictorial essay with a multimodality approach. J Anat 2010;217(6):633–45.

65. Nussbaum ED, Hosea TM, Sieler SD, et al. Prospective evaluation of syndesmotic ankle sprains without diastasis. Am J Sports Med 2001;29(1):31–5.

66. Beumer A, Swierstra BA, Mulder PGH. Clinical diagnosis of syndesmotic ankle instability: evaluation of stress tests behind the curtains. Acta Orthop Scand 2002;73(6):667–9.

67. Zalavras C, Thordarson D. Ankle syndesmotic injury. J Am Acad Orthop Surg 2007;15(6):330–9.

68. Ostrum RF, de Meo P, Subramanian R. A critical analysis of the anterior-posterior radiographic anatomy of the ankle syndesmosis. Foot Ankle Int 1995;16(3):128–31.

69. Pneumaticos SG, Noble PC, Chatziioannou SN, et al. The effects of rotation on radiographic evaluation of the tibiofibular syndesmosis. Foot Ankle Int 2002;23(2):107–11.

70. Ebraheim NA, Lu J, Yang H, et al. Radiographic and CT evaluation of tibiofibular syndesmotic diastasis: a cadaver study. Foot Ankle Int 1997;18(11):693–8.

71. Pakarinen H, Flinkkilä T, Ohtonen P, et al. Intraoperative assessment of the stability of the distal tibiofibular joint in supination-external rotation injuries of the ankle: sensitivity, specificity, and reliability of two clinical tests. J Bone Joint Surg Am 2011;93(22):2057–61.

72. Candal-Couto JJ, Burrow D, Bromage S, et al. Instability of the tibio-fibular syndesmosis: have we been pulling in the wrong direction? Injury 2004;35(8):814–8.

73. Leeds HC, Ehrlich MG. Instability of the distal tibiofibular syndesmosis after bimalleolar and trimalleolar ankle fractures. J Bone Joint Surg Am 1984;66:490–503.

74. Sagi HC, Shah AR, Sanders RW. The functional consequence of syndesmotic joint malreduction at a minimum 2-year follow-up. J Orthop Trauma 2012;26(7):439–43.

75. Kennedy JG, Soffe KE, Dalla Vedova P, et al. Evaluation of the syndesmotic screw in low Weber C ankle fractures. J Orthop Trauma 2000;14(5):359–66.

76. Chissell HR, Jones J. The influence of a diastasis screw on the outcome of Weber type-C ankle fractures. J Bone Joint Surg Br 1995;77(3):435–8.

77. Hunt KJ, Goeb Y, Behn AW, et al. Ankle joint contact loads and displacement with progressive syndesmotic injury. Foot Ankle Int 2015;36(9):1095–103.

78. Miller AN, Barei DP, Iaquinto JM, et al. Iatrogenic syndesmosis malreduction via clamp and screw placement. J Orthop Trauma 2013;27(2):100–6.

79. Phisitkul P, Ebinger T, Goetz J, et al. Forceps reduction of the syndesmosis in rotational ankle fractures: a cadaveric study. J Bone Joint Surg Am 2012; 94(24):2256–61.

80. Franke J, von Recum J, Suda AJ, et al. Intraoperative three-dimensional imaging in the treatment of acute unstable syndesmotic injuries. J Bone Joint Surg Am 2012;94(15):1386–90.

81. Koenig SJ, Tornetta P 3rd, Merlin G, et al. Can we tell if the syndesmosis is reduced using fluoroscopy? J Orthop Trauma 2015;29(9):e326–30.

82. Miller AN, Carroll EA, Parker RJ, et al. Direct visualization for syndesmotic stabilization of ankle fractures. Foot Ankle Int 2009;30(5):419–26.

83. Ruan Z, Luo C, Shi Z, et al. Intraoperative reduction of distal tibiofibular joint aided by three-dimensional fluoroscopy. Technol Health Care 2011;19(3):161–6.

84. Xie Y, Cai L, Deng Z, et al. Absorbable screws versus metallic screws for distal tibiofibular syndesmosis injuries: a meta-analysis. J Foot Ankle Surg 2015;54(4): 663–70.

85. Peek AC, Fitzgerald CE, Charalambides C. Syndesmosis screws: how many, what diameter, where and should they be removed? A literature review. Injury 2014;45(8):1262–7.

86. Wikerøy AKB, Høiness PR, Andreassen GS, et al. No difference in functional and radiographic results 8.4 years after quadricortical compared with tricortical syndesmosis fixation in ankle fractures. J Orthop Trauma 2010;24(1):17–23.

87. Høiness P, Strømsøe K. Tricortical versus quadricortical syndesmosis fixation in ankle fractures: a prospective, randomized study comparing two methods of syndesmosis fixation. J Orthop Trauma 2004;18(6):331–7.

88. Moore JA Jr, Shank JR, Morgan SJ, et al. Syndesmosis fixation: a comparison of three and four cortices of screw fixation without hardware removal. Foot Ankle Int 2006;27(8):567–72.

89. Beumer A, Campo MM, Niesing R, et al. Screw fixation of the syndesmosis: a cadaver model comparing stainless steel and titanium screws and three and four cortical fixation. Injury 2005;36(1):60–4.

90. Kukreti S, Faraj A, Miles JNV. Does position of syndesmotic screw affect functional and radiological outcome in ankle fractures? Injury 2005;36(9):1121–4.

91. Ahmad J, Raikin SM, Pour AE, et al. Bioabsorbable screw fixation of the syndesmosis in unstable ankle injuries. Foot Ankle Int 2009;30(2):99–105.

92. Hovis WD, Kaiser BW, Watson JT, et al. Treatment of syndesmotic disruptions of the ankle with bioabsorbable screw fixation. J Bone Joint Surg Am 2002;84(1): 26–31.

93. Kaukonen JP, Lamberg T, Korkala O, et al. Fixation of syndesmotic ruptures in 38 patients with a malleolar fracture: a randomized study comparing a metallic and a bioabsorbable screw. J Orthop Trauma 2005;19(6):392–5.

94. Thordarson DB, Samuelson M, Shepherd LE, et al. Bioabsorbable versus stainless steel screw fixation of the syndesmosis in pronation-lateral rotation ankle fractures: a prospective randomized trial. Foot Ankle Int 2001;22(4):335–8.

95. Sinisaari IP, Lüthje PMJ, Mikkonen RHM. Ruptured tibio-fibular syndesmosis: comparison study of metallic to bioabsorbable fixation. Foot Ankle Int 2002; 23(8):744–8.

96. Schepers T, van der Linden H, van Lieshout EM, et al. Technical aspects of the syndesmotic screw and their effect on functional outcome following acute distal tibiofibular syndesmosis injury. Injury 2014;45(4):775–9.

97. Darwish HH, Glisson RR, DeOrio JK. Compression screw fixation of the syndesmosis. Foot Ankle Int 2012;33(10):893–9.

98. Gardner R, Yousri T, Holmes F, et al. Stabilization of the syndesmosis in the Maisonneuve fracture–a biomechanical study comparing 2-hole locking plate and quadricortical screw fixation. J Orthop Trauma 2013;27(4):212–6.

99. Dunn WR, Easley ME, Parks BG, et al. An augmented fixation method for distal fibular fractures in elderly patients: a biomechanical evaluation. Foot Ankle Int 2004;25(3):128–31.

100. Mendelsohn ES, Hoshino CM, Harris TG, et al. The effect of obesity on early failure after operative syndesmosis injuries. J Orthop Trauma 2013;27(4):201–6.

101. Klitzman R, Zhao H, Zhang LQ, et al. Suture-button versus screw fixation of the syndesmosis: a biomechanical analysis. Foot Ankle Int 2010;31(1):69–75.

102. Teramoto A, Suzuki D, Kamiya T, et al. Comparison of different fixation methods of the suture-button implant for tibiofibular syndesmosis injuries. Am J Sports Med 2011;39(10):2226–32.

103. Laflamme M, Belzile EL, Bédard L, et al. A prospective randomized multicenter trial comparing clinical outcomes of patients treated surgically with a static or dynamic implant for acute ankle syndesmosis rupture. J Orthop Trauma 2015; 29(5):216–23.

104. Schepers T. Acute distal tibiofibular syndesmosis injury: a systematic review of suture-button versus syndesmotic screw repair. Int Orthop 2012;36(6): 1199–206.

105. Thornes B, Shannon F, Guiney AM, et al. Suture-button syndesmosis fixation: accelerated rehabilitation and improved outcomes. Clin Orthop Relat Res 2005;(431):207–12.

106. Peterson KS, Chapman WD, Hyer CF, et al. Maintenance of reduction with suture button fixation devices for ankle syndesmosis repair. Foot Ankle Int 2015;36(6): 679–84.

107. Dikos GD, Heisler J, Choplin RH, et al. Normal tibiofibular relationships at the syndesmosis on axial CT imaging. J Orthop Trauma 2012;26(7):433–8.

108. Knops SP, Kohn MA, Hansen EN, et al. Rotational malreduction of the syndesmosis: reliability and accuracy of computed tomography measurement methods. Foot Ankle Int 2013;34(10):1403–10.

109. Gifford PB, Lutz M. The tibiofibular line: an anatomical feature to diagnose syndesmosis malposition. Foot Ankle Int 2014;35(11):1181–6.

110. Egol KA, Pahk B, Walsh M, et al. Outcome after unstable ankle fracture: effect of syndesmotic stabilization. J Orthop Trauma 2010;24(1):7–11.

111. Hamid N, Loeffler BJ, Braddy W, et al. Outcome after fixation of ankle fractures with an injury to the syndesmosis: the effect of the syndesmosis screw. J Bone Joint Surg Br 2009;91(8):1069–73.

112. Manjoo A, Sanders DW, Tieszer C, et al. Functional and radiographic results of patients with syndesmotic screw fixation: implications for screw removal. J Orthop Trauma 2010;24(1):2–6.

113. Song DJ, Lanzi JT, Groth AT, et al. The effect of syndesmosis screw removal on the reduction of the distal tibiofibular joint: a prospective radiographic study. Foot Ankle Int 2014;35(6):543–8.

114. Schepers T. To retain or remove the syndesmotic screw: a review of literature. Arch Orthop Trauma Surg 2011;131(7):879–83.

115. Liu Q, Zhao G, Yu B, et al. Effects of inferior tibiofibular syndesmosis injury and screw stabilization on motion of the ankle: a finite element study. Knee Surg Sports Traumatol Arthrosc 2014. [Epub ahead of print].

116. Schepers T, van Lieshout EMM, de Vries MR, et al. Complications of syndesmotic screw removal. Foot Ankle Int 2011;32(11):1040–4.

117. Dattani R, Patnaik S, Kantak A, et al. Injuries to the tibiofibular syndesmosis. J Bone Joint Surg Br 2008;90(4):405–10.

118. Hsu YT, Wu CC, Lee WC, et al. Surgical treatment of syndesmotic diastasis: emphasis on effect of syndesmotic screw on ankle function. Int Orthop 2011; 35(3):359–64.

119. Pfeifer CG, Grechenig S, Frankewycz B, et al. Analysis of 213 currently used rehabilitation protocols in foot and ankle fractures. Injury 2015;46(Suppl 4): S51–7.

120. Lin CW, Donkers NA, Refshauge KM, et al. Rehabilitation for ankle fractures in adults. Cochrane Database Syst Rev 2012;(11):CD005595.

121. Richter J, Schulze W, Clasbrummel B, et al. The role of the tibiofibular syndesmotic and the deltoid ligaments in stabilizing Weber B type ankle joint fractures–an experimental investigation. Unfallchirurg 2003;106(5):359–66 [in German].

122. Hsu RY, Bariteau J. Management of ankle fractures. R I Med J (2013) 2013; 96(5):23–7.

123. Cimino W, Ichtertz D, Slabaugh P. Early mobilization of ankle fractures after open reduction and internal fixation. Clin Orthop Relat Res 1991;267:152–6.

124. Thomas G, Whalley H, Modi C. Early mobilization of operatively fixed ankle fractures: a systematic review. Foot Ankle Int 2009;30(7):666–74.

125. Papachristou G, Efstathopoulos N, Levidiotis C, et al. Early weight bearing after posterior malleolar fractures: an experimental and prospective clinical study. J Foot Ankle Surg 2003;42(2):99–104.

Foot and Ankle Injuries in Professional Soccer Players

Diagnosis, Treatment, and Expectations

Caio Nery, MD[a],*, Fernando Raduan, MD[b], Daniel Baumfeld, MD[c]

KEYWORDS

- Indoor soccer • Outdoor soccer • Soccer injuries • Injury prevention
- Sports rehabilitation

KEY POINTS

- Soccer injuries are frequent and have a high socioeconomic impact.
- Direct contact accounts for half of all injuries in both indoor and outdoor soccer.
- Ankle sprains are the most common foot and ankle injury in soccer players.
- Sixty percent of soccer players present anterior ankle impingement because repetitive ball impact may cause microtrauma to the anteromedial aspect of the ankle.
- An injury prevention program should include not only the players but also the trainer, responsible physician, and physical therapists.

INTRODUCTION

Soccer is one of the most popular sports in the world; it has a vivid and interesting history, and the players alternate between indoor and outdoor settings. Soccer injuries are frequent and have a high socioeconomic impact that probably exceeds US$30 billion per year.[1] The sport has undergone many changes in recent years, mainly because of increased physical demands. These changes have led to an increased injury risk. In Brazil, athletes are more prone to injury because of their extensive training and the large numbers of games they play.[2]

The incidence of injury in outdoor soccer has been reported in the literature, whereas there have been few studies on the injury rates of indoor soccer players. After the thigh, the feet and ankles are the most common locations for injury.[3] It is important

Disclosure: The authors have nothing to disclose.
a Foot and Ankle Clinic, UNIFESP – Escola Paulista de Medicina, São Paulo, São Paulo, Brazil;
b UNIFESP – Escola Paulista de Medicina, São Paulo, São Paulo, Brazil; c UFMG – Federal University of Minas Gerais, Belo Horizonte, Minas Gerais, Brazil
* Corresponding author. Hospital Israelita Albert Einstein. Av. Albert Einstein, 627 - Bloco A1 - sala 317, CEP 05652.000, São Paulo, Brazil
E-mail address: caionerymd@gmail.com

to identify the causes and types of injuries and the influence of preventive strategies and treatments.

INJURY DEFINITION AND TIME LOST

According to the National Athletic Injury Registration System of the United States, a soccer injury is defined as any physical complaint associated with soccer (received during training or match play) that limits athletic participation for at least a day after the day of onset.[4] The Union of European Football Associations Medical Committee injury definition is an injury that occurred during a scheduled training session or match that caused absence from the next training session or match.[5] It may also be appropriate to include injuries that cause the player to interrupt a training session or match, regardless of whether the player misses the next training session or match. This type of injury is particularly important at lower levels of the sport where training and matches are less frequent. These injuries could then be reported in a separate category as 0-day time-loss injuries.[6]

Injuries can be categorized into 4 levels of severity from the layoff times from soccer:

- Slight/minimal (0–3 days)
- Mild (4–7 days)
- Moderate (8–28 days)
- Severe (28 days)

A recurrent injury is defined as an injury of the same type and at the same site as an index injury occurring after a player's return to full participation from the index injury, and early recurrent injury is defined as a reinjury within 2 months after return to play.

EPIDEMIOLOGY

Analysis of soccer players after their career has ended has shown that they are more predisposed to ankle osteoarthritis than the general population. The high prevalence of osteoarthritis of the ankle among retired players (6%) suggests that there is an important need to identify the causes and mechanisms of foot and ankle injuries.[7]

The incidence of soccer injury has been investigated in several studies, and varies substantially depending on the definition of injury, characteristics of the investigated players, and research design. In general, the highest incidences of injury have been reported for players in the US professional league and the Icelandic national division league, and the lowest incidences have been reported for Dutch and Danish low-level players.[8–10] The incidence of match injuries is, on average, 4 to 6 times higher than the incidence of injuries that occur during training sessions.[8]

Regarding foot and ankle injuries, an epidemiologic study among 200 players of soccer on natural grass reported 66 severe ankle and foot problems (33%). The following injury mechanisms were reported[11]:

- Direct player-to-player contact (32.0%)
- Overuse (26.0%)
- Tripping on the grass (10.5%)
- Landing (7.5%)
- Jumping and jumping/landing (7.5%)
- Tackling (4.5%)
- Being tackled (4.5%)
- Shooting (3.0%)

- Kicking and kicking/shooting (3.0%)
- Sprinting (1.5%)

Most (59.0%) players had injuries of the right foot/ankle, and 79.0% were in the dominant extremity. The anatomic sites of injury were the ankle in 56.0%, hind foot in 30.0%, and midfoot in 14.0%. The most common injury mechanism for foot and ankle injuries in soccer has been reported to be direct contact in 58.0% of players, and in 59.0% in a study among professional English football players.[11,12]

Of all foot and ankle injuries, ankle sprains are the most common (80.0%), followed by bruises (9%–49.0%) and tendon lesions (2%–23.0%). Fractures are rare and account for only 1.0% of all ankle injuries in soccer.[13] Overall, soccer injuries are more frequent in older participants, whereas the incidence of injury in preadolescent players is low.[14] The incidence of foot and ankle injuries in elite soccer competition is estimated as between 3 and 9 injuries per 1000 player-hours of competition, and the dominant foot is most commonly injured.[15] Most injuries occur during competition rather than during training (2:1).[1,16,17]

Achilles tendon disorders account for 2.5% of all injuries and 3.8% of layoff times in male professional soccer, and the frequency varies considerably from country to country, perhaps because of the variation in sports traditions and popularity.[18] These disorders are more common in older players, and most (96%) disorders involve gradual onset of tendinopathy, with 4% involving acute partial or total ruptures. Not all databases classify Achilles tendinopathy and ruptures as foot and ankle injuries; sometimes, they are classified as lower leg injuries. The incidence of Achilles disorders is higher during the preseason than during the competitive season, and the median layoff time is 10 days for Achilles tendinopathies and 169 days for ruptures.[11]

RISK FACTORS

Several studies have described risk factors for injury in soccer players. Some studies recommend a differentiation between intrinsic (person-related) and extrinsic (environment-related) risk factors, which are defined as follows:

- Intrinsic risk factors are the individual biological or psychosocial characteristics, such as joint flexibility (including pathologic ligament laxity and muscle tightness), functional instability, previous injuries, and inadequate rehabilitation.
- Extrinsic risk factors include the amount of training and number of games played, climatic factors, pitch surface, playing field conditions (eg, dry, wet, uneven), equipment (eg, shin guards, taping, shoes), and the rules of the game and foul play.[19]

The most important extrinsic risk factor seems to be unfair play contact, which can cause approximately 23% to 33% of all injuries[19] (**Fig. 1**).

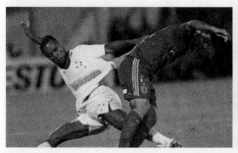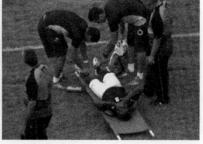

Fig. 1. Unfair play contact (*left*) and field player support (*right*).

In addition, inadequate preparation, such as insufficient training, inadequate warm-up, and incorrect or nonexistent ankle taping, has been shown to have an effect on the occurrence of injury. Intrinsic and extrinsic risk factors can partially influence each other, and therefore can increase the risk of injury or complaints.[8,19] However, Ekstrand and Gillquist[17] found that although 71.0% of the injuries could be related to risk factors, such as equipment, playing surface, and rules, 29.0% were considered to be caused by a chance event only.

Previous injuries and inadequate rehabilitation are the most important and well-established intrinsic risk factors for future soccer injury. Persistent symptoms may not only be an indicator of inadequate rehabilitation but also a precursor of future injury, a sign of overuse, or a sign of a minor injury.[20–22]

The importance of warm-up in the prevention of injury is well known. The lack of muscle strain injuries has been thought to be directly related to the initiation of a controlled warm-up and stretching program.[19]

INTERVENTIONS TO REDUCE THE RATE OF INJURY

A prevention program should include not only the players but also the trainer, responsible physician, and physical therapists (**Fig. 2**).

A theoretic framework for the prevention of sports injury involves 4 steps[8,23]:

- Step 1: establishing the extent of the sports injury problem
- Step 2: establishing the cause and mechanisms of injuries
- Step 3: introducing preventive measures
- Step 4: assessing the effectiveness of the preventive interventions by repeating step 1

COMMON TRAUMATIC INJURIES
Ankle Sprains

Ankle sprains represent 80% of all soccer injuries.[3] The most frequent mechanism of injury is inversion trauma, with the foot in various degrees of plantar flexion. Ankle ligament integrity provides mechanical stability of the joint, and functional stability is maintained by ankle proprioception provided by muscles, tendons, ligaments, and capsular innervation.[24]

After an inversion ankle trauma, injuries to the anterior talofibular ligament are the most common, followed by injuries to the calcaneal fibular ligament. The posterior talofibular ligament is usually uninjured unless there is a gross dislocation of the ankle.

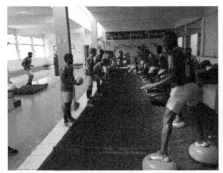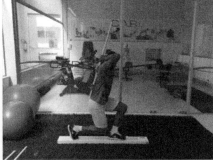

Fig. 2. Specific training of a professional soccer team to reduce the rate of injuries.

During the evaluation of a soccer player with an ankle sprain, any history of previous injuries should be considered. Soccer players with previous ankle sprain injuries are 4.9 times more likely to sustain a recurrent ankle sprain injury than are players without previous ankle sprains.[25] Some of the intrinsic risk factors involved in ankle injuries have been identified as previous sprains, cavus foot type, ankle instability, joint laxity, reduced lower extremity strength, and anatomic misalignment.[26]

The goal of treatment after an acute ankle sprain is to reduce the risk of chronic ankle instability and another ankle sprain. Eighty percent of all acute ankle sprains can achieve full recovery with conservative management, whereas 20% of them develop mechanical or functional instability, resulting in chronic ankle instability.[27]

An athlete with an acute lateral ankle ligament injury can be managed initially with rest, ice (cryotherapy), compression, and elevation, and the use of nonsteroidal anti-inflammatory drugs may be recommended for pain management.[28] Manual mobilizations of the ankle, ultrasonography therapy, laser therapy, and electrotherapy have been shown to add no value to the treatment. More than 2 weeks of immobilization in a lower leg cast is not an effective treatment strategy for patients who need fast rehabilitation.[29] However, a short period of immobilization can facilitate a rapid decrease in pain and swelling and can thus be helpful in the acute phase.[30] Thereafter, functional treatment is recommended, and as part of this functional approach the use of an ankle support is advocated. Exercise therapy should be recognized as being an essential element of the functional treatment of acute lateral ankle ligament injuries, but, in professional athletes, surgical treatment may be considered on an individual basis. Some investigators have recommended surgical intervention for athletes with higher objective and mechanical instability and with positive factures that could predispose for future sprains.[28] If surgery is chosen, it should begin with arthroscopy to assess the degree of ligament damage and accompanying injuries, such as syndesmotic injury or chondral/osteochondral lesions. The preferred method of reconstruction is direct anatomic ligament repair using a modified Broström-Gould procedure.[31]

The time needed to return to specific training or to game play depends on the severity of the main and associated lesions and the athlete's ability to perform the functional requirements of the sport. Because of the variability of injuries, there is no way to establish a rule. The back-to-game decision must be taken on an individual basis and can vary substantially from one athlete to another.

Muscular Injuries

Muscle injuries are common in soccer and represent up to 37.0% of all time-loss injuries at the men's professional level.[22] Ninety-two percent of all muscle injuries affect the 4 major muscle groups of the lower limbs: hamstrings (37.0%), adductors (23.0%), quadriceps (19.0%), and calf muscles (13.0%). A simple analysis showed that goalkeepers had a lower rate of calf injuries, whereas a higher rate was observed among older players and players with a previous calf injury. Calf injury rates increased during the competitive season and were evenly distributed between the left and right legs. Normally, this muscle injury is treated conservatively, and the time lost to play is 15 days on average.[32]

Tendon Lesions

The Achilles is the most common tendon injured in soccer players, but the peroneal tendons, posterior tibial tendon, flexor halluces longus tendon, and posterior tibial tendon can also be affected.[11] Achilles tendon rupture is frequent among soccer players; 9 of 100,000 Achilles tendon ruptures can be attributed to soccer.[33] The risk for rupture is higher with increased training intensity and is 3 times higher before than during the competitive season.[12] A rupture normally occurs in its typical location; approximately 2 to 6 cm proximal to the insertion, where vascularity and healing potential are low. Patients can present a palpable gap in the tendon and an insufficient Achilles tendon. In this type of patient, an MRI scan can be helpful in addition to clinical diagnosis for the identification of degeneration of fatty infiltration in the proximal muscle. Conservative treatment is not recommended in high-performing athletes.[33] The preferred treatment is a miniopen or percutaneous technique with accelerated rehabilitation.

Bruises and Contusions

Contusions and bruises tend to be minor injuries for soccer players. Rarely do severe injuries and complications occur because of bruising or contusions. The shins and thighs are the most commonly affected sites.[34] Bruises are typically acquired by a player's contact with an opponent or with the ground. Pain, swelling, and reduced muscle functions are typical symptoms. Initial examinations can detect variable amounts of swelling, hematomas, and local pain. Fractures are rare, but need to be ruled out by clinical examination and radiographs. Initial treatment includes painkillers, ice, and compression, with restriction from activity depending on the severity of the injury. The intensity of physical therapy must be consistent with the severity of the symptoms; careful stretching of the affected muscle followed by gradual strengthening and progressive functional activity is needed. Before returning to play, full range of motion, symmetric strength, and the ability to perform the functional requirements of soccer have to be reached.[31] Complications and disabilities are rare, but muscle tears and ruptures, compartment syndrome, and myositis ossificans can occur.

Osteochondral Lesions

Osteochondral lesions of the talus can lead to mechanical pain and swelling that precludes resumption of sports activities. Acute lesions caused by ankle sprains or ankle fractures can occur. The clinical symptoms of osteochondral talar lesions include deep and nonlocalized pain, recurrent synovitis, joint balance alterations, and loose bodies. The symptoms are not specific to this condition and, because these lesions are uncommon, they can be mistaken for acute or chronic ankle sprains. For this reason, with professional soccer players, it is important to perform extensive conventional radiography and MRI. To improve surgical planning, computed tomography (CT) or single-photon emission CT–CT is recommended (**Fig. 3**).

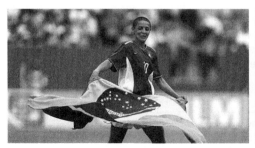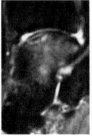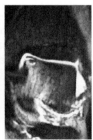

Fig. 3. Osteochondral lesion (*middle, right*) in a female soccer player and her celebration (*left*), 2 years after the treatment, after winning third place in the 1999 FIFA Female World Cup.

Surgical intervention depends on the size and location of the lesion:

- Acute lesions: arthroscopic debridement, microfracturing, or fragment fixation
- Chronic lesions: 1-step repair (microfractures, osteochondral autograft transfer system) or 2-step repair (osteochondral transplantation)[35]

Additional healing augmentation with platelet-rich plasma or hyaluronic acid has been reported to improve the treatment of this lesion.[36,37] The ability to return to the same level of sports practice as before the injury is a good indication that the lesion has satisfactorily resolved. Some investigators have stated that it is important that the healing of these lesions restores the normal joint biomechanics, and sometimes a calcaneus osteotomy or supramalleolar osteotomy may be required.[35]

Fractures

Soccer involves intense body-to-body contact during matches, and fractures caused by energy transfer from an opponent's lower leg may result. The incidence of fractures in soccer has been reported to range from 1% to 9.7% of all injuries.[38] Seventy-five percent of all fractures occur during competitive matches.[39]

Of all lower leg fractures, ankle fractures are the most common (36%), followed by fractures of the foot (33%) and the tibia (22%). Dvorak and colleagues[19] found a 2% incidence rate for fractures in outdoor soccer and an 8% rate for indoor soccer. Gender, recreational level, and age are important risk factors for lower leg fractures. Because of its low incidence, the authors found no data on the exact classification and morphology of ankle fractures among soccer players. Overall, supination and external rotation are the most common mechanisms underlying ankle fractures in sports. Fracture treatment follows the basic classic principles, but, in athletes, diagnostic ankle arthroscopy at the time of open reduction with internal fixation is a powerful tool for uncovering osteochondral lesions. Untreated acute osteochondral lesions have a tendency not to heal properly and become chronic lesions, which causes pain and inhibits playing ability.

Another traumatic injury in soccer is the fifth metatarsal fracture. A recent study showed that this rare type of injury was associated with a high rate of healing problems in soccer players.[40] Further findings of this study were that almost all fractures in soccer players were located at the base of the bone and that avulsions were very rare. Most fifth metatarsal fractures are stress fractures and mainly occur in young players. In total, 54.0% of fifth metatarsal fractures were classified as Torg type II (stress fractures), and 46% were classified as Torg type I (acute type). Because of frequent healing problems, which might be explained by the stress nature of the injury, the investigators recommend surgical treatment as a primary management. These fractures healed faster after surgical treatment than after conservative treatment (75.0% vs 33.0%, respectively; $P<.05$)[40] **(Fig. 4)**.

COMMON NONTRAUMATIC INJURIES
Tendon

Achilles tendon complaints are most common among soccer players. The potential causes of a painful Achilles tendon are tendinitis, midportion tendinopathy, insertion tendinopathy, malalignment of the ankle joint, or Haglund deformity. All of these injuries may be caused by overuse, training errors, medications, or personal physical predisposition. The important risk factors for Achilles tendon overuse injuries are hard ground, resumption of training after a break, poor footwear, increased intensity of training and running, and loss of ankle dorsiflexion. Therefore, increased attention to players' plantar flexor strength and amount of dorsiflexion excursion (an intrinsic

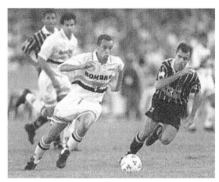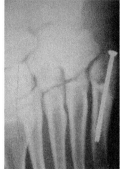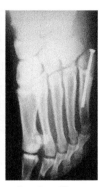

Fig. 4. Fifth metatarsal stress fractures (*middle, right*) treated with a screw in a Brazilian professional soccer player (*left*).

risk factor) may prevent such injuries.[12,41] All tendinopathies should be treated conservatively initially with eccentric exercises, therapeutic ultrasonography, and adaptation of training intensity and choice of shoes. If conservative treatment fails, which is not common, surgery may be necessary.[31]

Anterior Impingement

Anterior ankle impingement syndrome caused by anterior osteophytes is related to recurrent ball impact, which can be regarded as repetitive microtrauma to the anteromedial aspect of the ankle.[42] It is estimated that approximately 60% of soccer players may present with this syndrome.[31] Anterior pain with ankle hyperdorsiflexion, restriction of dorsiflexion, and swelling is a classic presentation. The cause of the pain can be either soft tissue or bony impingement (**Fig. 5**).

Lateral ankle radiographs reveal osteophytes on the anterior tibia and talar neck (kissing osteophytes). The diagnostic value of an oblique radiograph as an addition to a lateral radiograph has been shown. When the lateral radiograph was combined with an oblique anteromedial radiograph, the sensitivity and specificity of the method was high.[43]

The treatment of lesions that fail to respond to conservative treatment is arthroscopic or open debridement. It is important to consider the possibility of coexisting instabilities of the ankle joint. Results of ankle arthroscopic soft tissue debridement and osteophyte resection are good, satisfaction is high (>94.0–98.0%), and the rate of major complications is only 1.0%.[44]

Posterior Impingement

Posterior ankle impingement syndrome (PAIS) is a clinical disorder defined as a painful limitation of ankle range of motion; more specifically, forced plantarflexion, either

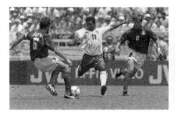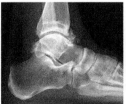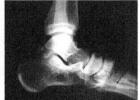

Fig. 5. Preoperative view (*middle*) and postoperative treatment (*right*) of anterior bone impingement in a Brazilian former professional soccer player (*left*).

acute secondary to a traumatic injury or chronic, caused by repeated stress. There are several possible causes of PAIS, including soft tissue lesions; Achilles or flexor hallucis longus tendinopathies; retrocalcaneal bursitis; os trigonum syndrome; and bone, osteochondral, or neurovascular lesions that involve the Stieda process and fractures. Among soccer players, the ankle is subjected to a great variety of chronic biomechanical forces from jumping, spinning around, and kicking a ball. PAIS symptoms arise more commonly when the soccer player sprints or hits the ball, which results in forced plantarflexion of the ankle. Clinical suspicions can be confirmed by plain radiography of the ankle in anteroposterior and lateral views and an MRI scan to rule out other causes. Conservative treatment and modification of sports activities are the first-line treatments and include rest, ice, antiinflammatory drugs, immobilization (bracing to limit plantarflexion), and physical therapy. Approximately 60.0% of conservatively treated athletes show improvement of their symptoms. Operative treatment is only recommended when players do not experience any improvement or even worsen with conservative treatment; in such cases, the preferred approach is endoscopic surgery.[45,46]

SPECIAL FEATURES
Indoor Soccer

Indoor soccer is an increasingly popular sport that has attracted more and more followers all over the world. In Brazil, indoor soccer is one of the most commonly played sports and is played by more than 12 million people, according to the Futsal Brazilian Confederation.[47] Indoor soccer is associated with an approximately 2-times higher injury rate than outdoor soccer tournaments.[48] Such a difference can be attributed to the nature of the game, and could be associated with the high speed of the movements, the smaller size of the field, and differences in the surface, which typically result in a higher number of collisions and sprains. Most indoor soccer injuries are caused by direct contact, and ankle sprains and contusions are the most common type, ranging from 23.0% to 29.0% and 23.0% to 23.5% of all injuries, respectively.[49] The high incidence of ankle injuries relative to those associated with outdoor soccer's grass may be attributed to the rubberized and more adherent surfaces of the floors used in indoor soccer.

Treatment of indoor soccer injuries follows the same principles as are used to treat outdoor injuries.

Beach Soccer

Barefoot beach soccer is played by thousands of people in South America. It is similar to indoor soccer in terms of techniques and playing time, but the characteristics of the sand court make beach soccer a distinctive sport. Thus, it must involve different types of injuries with different mechanisms. Most of the injuries in beach soccer players occur in their feet and toes (36.4%), followed by the Achilles tendon as the second most prevalent injury (18.2%). Forty-four percent of all foot injuries have occurred in toes. Among the toes, the hallux alone accounts for 11.1% of foot injuries. This injury incidence may be caused by the lack of any footwear or shin guards worn by beach soccer players. Injuries occur more often during competitions (72.7%) than during training (27.3%). Most foot injuries are caused by hitting the ball (55.6%) and blocking (22.2%).[50] Despite the common injuries that can occur in all soccer athletes, on all types of surfaces, there is a specific clinical syndrome characterized by progressive pain and swelling in the dominant (kicking side) hallux metatarsophalangeal (MTP) or interphalangeal (IP) joints of barefoot beach soccer players that can lead to an osteochondral injury of the hallux (**Fig. 6**). The mechanism of injury is repetitive

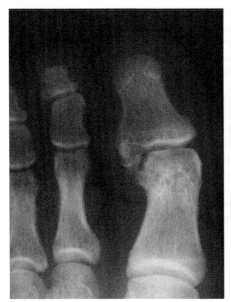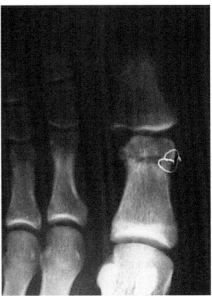

Fig. 6. Osteochondral injury of the hallux in a beach soccer player: Initial image (*left*); Post-operative image (*right*).

hyperextension or hyperflexion with repetitive trauma of the hallux MTP or IP joints. The end result can be acute fracture or stress fracture at the lateral or medial margins of the joints. Radiographic evaluation can show a marginal, often sclerotic, bony fragment within the involved symptomatic MTP or IP joint. MRI can reveal sclerosis of the free bony fragment. When a symptomatic bony fragment is identified within the MTP or IP joints of the hallux, simple excision has been reported to predictably relieve symptoms.[51]

PREVENTION

Several investigators have discussed possibilities for prevention of soccer injuries; the most accepted are listed here.[4,5,8,12,19,23,26,52]

- Warm-up with more emphasis on stretching
- Regular cool-down
- Adequate rehabilitation with sufficient recovery time
- Proprioceptive training (**Fig. 7**)
- Protective equipment
- Good playing field conditions
- Adherence to the existing rules

FUTURE DIRECTIONS

Lower extremity injuries are common in both indoor and outdoor soccer, and should be targeted for injury prevention strategies. Specifically, ankle sprains account for the greatest proportion of injuries, by specific injury type, in both indoor and outdoor soccer. In addition, direct contact accounts for half of all injuries in both indoor and outdoor soccer. Body contact regulations and enforcement should be given consideration for further investigation.

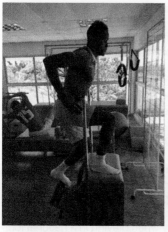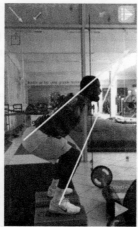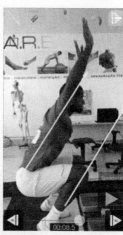

Fig. 7. Rehabilitation program for injured professional soccer players. Rehabilitation program for body balance (*Left picture*). Wrong body posture during the exercise - line should not cross during the movement (*Middle picture*). Correct body position - parallel lines (*Right picture*).

REFERENCES

1. Wong P, Hong Y. Soccer injury in the lower extremities. Br J Sports Med 2005;39: 473–82.
2. Arliani GG, Belangero PS, Runco JL, et al. The Brazilian Football Association (CBF) model for epidemiological studies on professional soccer player injuries. Clinics (Sao Paulo) 2011;66:1707–12.
3. Giza E, Fuller C, Junge A, et al. Mechanisms of foot and ankle injuries in soccer. Am J Sports Med 2003;31:550–4.
4. van Mechelen W, Hlobil H, Kemper HC. Incidence, severity, aetiology and prevention of sports injuries. A review of concepts. Sports Med 1992;14:82–99.
5. Ekstrand J. A training program for the prevention of injuries to reduce soccer injuries by 75 per cent. Nord Med 1982;97:164–5 [in Swedish].
6. Hägglund M, Waldén M, Bahr R, et al. Methods for epidemiological study of injuries to professional football players: developing the UEFA model. Br J Sports Med 2005;39:340–6.
7. Larsen E, Jensen PK, Jensen PR. Long-term outcome of knee and ankle injuries in elite football. Scand J Med Sci Sports 1999;9:285–9.
8. Junge A, Dvorak J. Soccer injuries: a review on incidence and prevention. Sports Med 2004;34:929–38.
9. Arnason A, Gudmundsson A, Dahl HA, et al. Soccer injuries in Iceland. Scand J Med Sci Sports 1996;6:40–5.
10. Morgan BE, Oberlander MA. An examination of injuries in major league soccer. The inaugural season. Am J Sports Med 2001;29:426–30.
11. Oztekin HH, Boya H, Ozcan O, et al. Foot and ankle injuries and time lost from play in professional soccer players. Foot (Edinb) 2009;19:22–8.
12. Woods C, Hawkins R, Hulse M, et al. The Football Association Medical Research Programme: an audit of injuries in professional football: an analysis of ankle sprains. Br J Sports Med 2003;37:233–8.
13. Fong DT, Hong Y, Chan LK, et al. A systematic review on ankle injury and ankle sprain in sports. Sports Med 2007;37:73–94.

14. Sullivan JA, Gross RH, Grana WA, et al. Evaluation of injuries in youth soccer. Am J Sports Med 1980;8:325–7.
15. Hawkins RD, Hulse MA, Wilkinson C, et al. The association football medical research programme: an audit of injuries in professional football. Br J Sports Med 2001;35:43–7.
16. Hawkins RD, Fuller CW. A prospective epidemiological study of injuries in four English professional football clubs. Br J Sports Med 1999;33:196–203.
17. Ekstrand J, Gillquist J. Soccer injuries and their mechanisms: a prospective study. Med Sci Sports Exerc 1983;15:267–70.
18. Kannus P, Natri A. Etiology and pathophysiology of tendon ruptures in sports. Scand J Med Sci Sports 1997;7:107–12.
19. Dvorak J, Junge A. Football injuries and physical symptoms. A review of the literature. Am J Sports Med 2000;28:S3–9.
20. Baumhauer JF, Alosa DM, Renstrom AF, et al. A prospective study of ankle injury risk factors. Am J Sports Med 1995;23:564–70.
21. Ekstrand J, Waldén M, Hägglund M. Risk for injury when playing in a national football team. Scand J Med Sci Sports 2004;14:34–8.
22. Hägglund M, Waldén M, Ekstrand J. Risk factors for lower extremity muscle injury in professional soccer: the UEFA Injury Study. Am J Sports Med 2013;41:327–35.
23. Klügl M, Shrier I, McBain K, et al. The prevention of sport injury: an analysis of 12,000 published manuscripts. Clin J Sport Med 2010;20:407–12.
24. Hintermann B. Biomechanics of the unstable ankle joint and clinical implications. Med Sci Sports Exerc 1999;31:S459–69.
25. Kofotolis ND, Kellis E, Vlachopoulos SP. Ankle sprain injuries and risk factors in amateur soccer players during a 2-year period. Am J Sports Med 2007;35:458–66.
26. Inklaar H. Soccer injuries. II: aetiology and prevention. Sports Med 1994;18: 81–93.
27. Chan KW, Ding BC, Mroczek KJ. Acute and chronic lateral ankle instability in the athlete. Bull NYU Hosp Jt Dis 2011;69:17–26.
28. Kerkhoffs GM, Van Dijk CN. Acute lateral ankle ligament ruptures in the athlete: the role of surgery. Foot Ankle Clin 2013;18:215–8.
29. Kerkhoffs GM, Rowe BH, Assendelft WJ, et al. Immobilisation for acute ankle sprain. A systematic review. Arch Orthop Trauma Surg 2001;121:462–71.
30. Lamb SE, Marsh JL, Hutton JL, et al. Mechanical supports for acute, severe ankle sprain: a pragmatic, multicentre, randomised controlled trial. Lancet 2009;373: 575–81.
31. Valderrabano V, Barg A, Paul J, et al. Foot and ankle injuries in professional soccer players. Sports Orthopaedics and Traumatology 2014;30:98–105.
32. Ekstrand J, Hagglund M, Walden M. Epidemiology of muscle injuries in professional football (soccer). Am J Sports Med 2011;39:1226–32.
33. Cretnik A, Frank A. Incidence and outcome of rupture of the Achilles tendon. Wiener klinische Wochenschrift 2004;116(Suppl 2):33–8.
34. Tucker AM. Common soccer injuries. Diagnosis, treatment and rehabilitation. Sports Med 1997;23:21–32.
35. Valderrabano V, Barg A, Alattar A, et al. Osteochondral lesions of the ankle joint in professional soccer players: treatment with autologous matrix-induced chondrogenesis. Foot Ankle Spec 2014;7:522–8.
36. Smyth NA, Murawski CD, Haleem AM, et al. Establishing proof of concept: platelet-rich plasma and bone marrow aspirate concentrate may improve cartilage repair following surgical treatment for osteochondral lesions of the talus. World J Orthopedics 2012;3:101–8.

37. Hall MP, Band PA, Meislin RJ, et al. Platelet-rich plasma: current concepts and application in sports medicine. J Am Acad Orthop Surg 2009;17:602–8.
38. Engstrom B, Johansson C, Tornkvist H. Soccer injuries among elite female players. Am J Sports Med 1991;19:372–5.
39. Vanlommel L, Vanlommel J, Bollars P, et al. Incidence and risk factors of lower leg fractures in Belgian soccer players. Injury 2013;44:1847–50.
40. Ekstrand J, van Dijk CN. Fifth metatarsal fractures among male professional footballers: a potential career-ending disease. Br J Sports Med 2013;47:754–8.
41. Mahieu NN, Witvrouw E, Stevens V, et al. Intrinsic risk factors for the development of Achilles tendon overuse injury: a prospective study. Am J Sports Med 2006;34: 226–35.
42. Tol JL, Slim E, van Soest AJ, et al. The relationship of the kicking action in soccer and anterior ankle impingement syndrome. A biomechanical analysis. Am J Sports Med 2002;30:45–50.
43. Tol JL, Verhagen RA, Krips R, et al. The anterior ankle impingement syndrome: diagnostic value of oblique radiographs. Foot Ankle Int 2004;25:63–8.
44. Parma A, Buda R, Vannini F, et al. Arthroscopic treatment of ankle anterior bony impingement: the long-term clinical outcome. Foot Ankle Int 2014;35:148–55.
45. Lopez Valerio V, Seijas R, Alvarez P, et al. Endoscopic repair of posterior ankle impingement syndrome due to os trigonum in soccer players. Foot Ankle Int 2015;36:70–4.
46. Ribbans WJ, Ribbans HA, Cruickshank JA, et al. The management of posterior ankle impingement syndrome in sport: a review. Foot Ankle Surg 2015;21:1–10.
47. Ribeiro RN, Costa LOP. Análise epidemiológica de lesões no futebol de salão durante o XV Campeonato Brasileiro de Seleções Sub 20. Rev Bras Med Esporte 2006;12:1–5.
48. Junge A, Dvorak J, Graf-Baumann T, et al. Football injuries during FIFA tournaments and the Olympic Games, 1998-2001: development and implementation of an injury-reporting system. Am J Sports Med 2004;32:80s–9s.
49. Lindenfeld TN, Schmitt DJ, Hendy MP, et al. Incidence of injury in indoor soccer. Am J Sports Med 1994;22:364–71.
50. Mina H, Faezeh Z, Leila Z. Incidence and mechanisms of injuries in female beach soccer players. Ann Biol Res 2012;3:3508.
51. Altman A, Nery C, Sanhudo A, et al. Osteochondral injury of the hallux in beach soccer players. Foot Ankle Int 2008;29:919–21.
52. Gabbe BJ, Finch CF, Wajswelner H, et al. Predictors of lower extremity injuries at the community level of Australian football. Clin J Sport Med 2004;14:56–63.

Recent Advances in Egypt for Treatment of Talar Osteochondral Lesions

Amgad M. Haleem, MD, PhD[a,b,*], Mostafa M. AbouSayed, MD[b,c],
Mohammed Gomaa, MD[b]

KEYWORDS

- Osteochondral lesions • Talus • Articular cartilage • Repair • Reconstruction
- Tissue engineering

KEY POINTS

- Treatment of osteochondral lesions (OCLs) of the talus among other weightbearing joints of the lower extremity remains a most challenging arena in orthopedic surgery.
- The basis of marrow stimulation gave way to novel tissue engineering techniques involving various cell niches, growth factors, and scaffolds.
- This article highlights current state-of-the-art techniques and reviews the literature on recent advances in articular cartilage repair using various novel tissue engineering approaches, including various scaffolds, growth factors, and cell niches; which include chondrocytes and culture expanded bone marrow-derived mesenchymal stem cells.

 Video content accompanies this article at http://www.foot.theclinics.com

INTRODUCTION

Osteochondral lesions (OCLs) of the talus encompass several synonyms that define a lesion of any origin that involves the articular surface of the talar dome with the underlying subchondral bone. These include osteochondral defects, osteocartilaginous bodies, osteochondritis dissecans, early avascular necrosis, transchondral fractures, and intra-articular fragmentary fragments. These lesions are commonly associated with ankle injuries. They have been shown to occur in up to 50% of ankle sprains

---

The authors have nothing to disclose.
[a] Department of Orthopedic Surgery, Oklahoma University College of Medicine Health Sciences Center, Oklahoma City, OK, USA; [b] Department of Orthopedic Surgery, Kasr Al-Ainy Hospital, Cairo University School of Medicine, Saray El-Manial Street, El-Manial, Cairo 12411, Egypt; [c] Department of Orthopedic Surgery, Albany Medical College, 1367 Washington Avenue, Albany, NY 12206, USA
* Corresponding author. Department of Orthopedic Surgery, Oklahoma University College of Medicine Health Sciences Center, 920 Stanton L Young Blvd, WP 1380, Oklahoma City, OK 73104.
E-mail addresses: haleem@kasralainy.edu.eg; amgad-haleem@ouhsc.edu

Foot Ankle Clin N Am 21 (2016) 405–420
http://dx.doi.org/10.1016/j.fcl.2016.01.010
foot.theclinics.com

and fractures.[1] Although the predominant cause remains traumatic,[2] several atraumatic causes have been described in patients without a history of trauma. Such theories include spontaneous necrosis,[3,4] embolic disease, alcohol abuse, endocrine abnormalities,[5] unstable ankle ligaments,[6] and potential congenital or hereditary factors.[7,8]

Treatment of osteochondral lesions (OCLs) of the talus, among other weightbearing joints of the lower extremity, has evolved from palliative treatment, such as debridement and lavage or abrasion chondroplasty, to what may be called the 3 "R" paradigm: reconstruction, repair, and replacement. Reconstruction involves reattachment of OCLs by biodegradable fixation devices and/or reconstructing the contour of the articular surface by autologous or allogenous osteochondral grafts. Repair includes the formation of reparative tissue by marrow stimulation techniques, namely microfracture (MF). The basis of marrow stimulation gave way to novel tissue engineering techniques involving various cell niches, growth factors, and scaffolds. Replacement involves the final stage of joint salvage by partial or total replacement of the articular surfaces with metal prosthesis. Given the finite lifespan of these prosthesis and their infeasible use in the younger active population with high demands, evolution of tissue engineering modalities for cartilage repair has given way to a wide array of techniques that aim at restoring the complex hyaline nature of articular cartilage.

Currently, cartilage tissue engineering has 3 cornerstones. The first is a cell niche with chondrogenic potential that enables proliferation and differentiation into mature chondrocytes. Second, a scaffold is needed that is chondroconductive and/or chondroinductive. Chondroconductivity is defined as providing a structural framework for cartilage growth, whereas chondroinductivity involves the internal ability of the scaffold to provide chondrogenic factors that stimulate cartilage formation and induction of stem cells and/or chondrocytes down a hyaline cartilage-forming lineage. The third cornerstone involves growth factors that need to be introduced to stimulate the chondrogenic cellular pathway with subsequent production of a hyaline extracellular matrix with predominant type II collagen and aggrecan.

This article highlights the current state-of-the-art techniques in cartilage tissue engineering and regeneration, with special emphasis on clinical applications and a brief literature review. The main focus is on various clinically available scaffolds, growth factors, and cell niches; namely chondrocytes and culture-expanded bone marrow-derived (BM) mesenchymal stem cell (MSCs), with which the authors had a relatively extensive experience in Egypt.

DECISION-MAKING IN MANAGEMENT OF OSTEOCHONDRAL DEFECTS

Given the abundant options of surgical treatment of OCLs of the talar dome, the approach to cartilage tissue regeneration strategies should be tailored to each individual. The most important factors to consider in the management of OCLs are patient-specific and lesion-specific. Patient-specific factors include age, body mass index (BMI), activity levels, functional demands, and ability to comply with rehabilitation. Older patients are not candidates for autologous cell implantation techniques because cell senescence is a concerning factor, even with mesenchymal stem cell populations that were proven to undergo senescence.[9,10] Systemic inflammatory and immunosuppressive disorders negate the use of tissue engineering techniques involving implantation of live or culture-expanded cells. The inflammatory process associated with these diseases hinders chondrogenic differentiation of such implanted cell populations. Lesion-specific factors include defect cause, size, site, containment,[11] condition of the surrounding cartilage, and extent of involvement of the subchondral bone[12]; all of which significantly contribute to the decision-making paradigm.[13]

BONE MARROW STIMULATION: MICROFRACTURE

MF has been established as the standard of care for treating small lesions of the talar dome due to its technical simplicity, single-stage nature, and cost-effectiveness. It relies on making 2 mm perforations in the subchondral bone to produce a dilute mesenchymal blood clot through the recruitment of local BM-MSCs. Although the general consensus was that MF was reserved for OCLs that do not exceed 15 mm^2,[11,13–15] recent evidence has reconsidered this critical size and recommended the cut-off size of OCLs to be treated with MF is not exceed 10 mm^2 due to the declining clinical outcome scores and mechanical changes of the ankle joint in 10 to 15 mm^2 size lesions.[16] It is thought that the small concentration of BM-MSCs in the mesenchymal blood clot formed at the base of the MF defect does not support a robust chondrogenic response in the challenging mechanical environment of a large OCL. This, in addition to several other factors, may hinder the results of MF in defects larger than 10 mm^2. These factors include, first, that the potential violation of the subchondral bone through MF may lead to enchondral ossification and increased oxygen tension from the inflow of vascular marrow. Both of these may impede effective chondrogenesis.[17] Second, cell senescence, including senescence of local BM-MSCs, is believed to weaken their chondrogenic potential and thus affect the quality of the repair tissue in situ.[18] These factors result in repair tissue that is predominantly of fibrocartilaginous nature, with inferior mechanical properties and questionable longevity, as evidenced from studies of MF in the knee.[19,20] In light of all the aforementioned, the following guidelines have been recommended for MF to achieve successful outcomes of the procedure: age less than 40 years,[21] lower BMI (< 30),[11] small-size lesions (< 1.0 cm^2) in the talus,[16] and preoperative duration of symptoms fewer than 12 months.[22]

Retrograde Drilling

In early phases of OCLs, namely osteochondritis dissecans and OCLs with large subchondral cysts, the pathologic state primarily involves the subchondral bone with an occasional intact cartilaginous cap. Such lesions, in addition to lesions that might not be readily accessible through standard arthroscopic portals, may be managed by retrograde drilling. This process induces decompression and revascularization of the subchondral edema and cysts with new bone formation, while protecting the unviolated cartilage surface. Drilling can then be augmented with retrograde filling of the drill sites with cancellous bone graft or bone graft substitutes to support the subchondral bone and promote bone healing. The greatest challenge with this technique, however, is the difficulty targeting the lesion. Therefore, intraoperative fluoroscopy is usually used to aid in visualizing the subchondral lesion. This is sometimes hindered by the limited 2-dimensional nature of the intraoperative fluoroscopic image and incomplete visualization of the relatively hypodense pathologic subchondral lesion. Recent results have shown favorable outcomes with retrograde drilling with clinical outcomes improvement and MRI evidence of complete healing of the subchondral bone,[23] with success rates in one study reaching 88%.[24]

OSTEOCHONDRAL AUTOGRAFT TRANSPLANTATION

Osteochondral autograft transplantation (OAT) encompasses both OAT and mosaicplasty. OAT involves transplantation of a single osteochondral plug, whereas mosaicplasty entails implantation of multiple small cylindrical plugs, usually harvested from the patient's nonweightbearing articular surface of the femur. OAT or mosaicplasty have the major advantage of reconstructing the articular surface with hyaline cartilage in a single-stage procedure. It also effectively addresses OCLs with deep subchondral cyst involvement because it replaces the whole diseased OCL. A major disadvantage of the procedure is donor site morbidity at the graft harvest site. Another major disadvantage is the need for performing the procedure via an open miniarthrotomy with potential need for osteotomizing the medial malleolus, fibula, or the anterior tibial plafond to access the lesion. Finally, the graft-host interface may present a challenge due to fibrocartilage tissue filling the interface between the plug or plugs and native cartilage, which has inferior mechanical properties, limited quality, and has been shown to allow fluid ingress to the subchondral bone leading to subsequent subchondral cyst formation.[25] Although the senior author (AH) has reported that the results of double-plug OAT (mosaicplasty) did not show inferior clinical or radiological outcomes compared with results with a single-plug OAT, both groups showed abnormal subchondral bone signal intensity (edema or cyst).[26] This has been the point of continuous investigation by the same author, who subsequently reported on a novel technique in vitro that may prevent synovial fluid ingress and subchondral bone cyst formation through sealing of the graft-host interface by chemical tissue bonding, which might have future applications in the clinical setting.[27]

Although usually reserved for reconstruction of large-sized cartilage lesions beyond the critical size identified for MF (10 mm^2), single-plug OAT may be indicated for smaller size OCLs (8 mm) with deep bony involvement and subchondral cyst formation, or as a salvage open procedure after failed MF in such lesions. However, the condition of the articular surface of the patient's donor knee joint, particularly in the relatively older patient population, must be carefully assessed because the presence of degenerative changes in the knee is a contraindication to the procedure and indicates an alternative treatment modality needs to be used. Concerns about the differences in radius of curvature and thickness between knee donor and ankle recipient sites, as well as graft proudness or subsidence relative to the surface of surrounding ankle cartilage after implantation, may result in altered contact pressures, leading to negative implications on graft survival.[28] Finally, gentle impaction of the graft into its bed is crucial to avoid compromising chondrocyte viability at the surface of the graft.[29,30]

AUTOLOGOUS CHONDROCYTE IMPLANTATION

Autologous chondrocyte implantation (ACI) was originally described as a 2-stage procedure in the first-generation procedure. This involved arthroscopic retrieval of cartilage from nonweightbearing areas of the knee, followed by in vitro culture expansion of the harvested cartilage after digestion of the matrix and isolation of its chondrocytes. This was followed by a second-stage procedure for implantation of these culture-expanded chondrocytes by injecting them while in suspension under a periosteal flap that was harvested from the proximal tibia and sutured to the edges of the OCL, and then sealed by fibrin glue. Disadvantages of first-generation ACI included donor site morbidity to the knee articular surface and periosteum harvest site, requirement of 2 surgeries, nonarthroscopic nature of the second-stage arthrotomy, damage to the edges of the OCL from suturing the periosteal flap, uneven distribution of the cell suspension within the defect, potential cell leakage, periosteal graft delamination, and hypertrophy.[31]

To avoid these limitations, second-generation ACI was introduced. This procedure involved seeding the cultured chondrocytes on various scaffolds in vitro before the second-stage implantation to ensure homogenous cellular distribution on implantation in the OCL, together with easier fixation on the scaffold to the base of the cartilaginous defect by fibrin glue in a dry, all-arthroscopic technique. The primary scaffold initially used in second-generation ACI was a porcine collagen I/III membrane. This was followed by introduction of other scaffolds, including bovine collagen,[32] hyaluronic acid–based scaffolds, and polyglycolic–polylactic acid (PLG/PLA) scaffolds.[33] The PLG/PLA scaffold was subsequently abandoned because its degradative products produced an acidic environment that would hinder chondrocyte growth.

Further evolution of ACI led to the introduction of the third-generation procedure in which the chondrocytes were culture-expanded on 3-dimensional matrices to maintain their chondrogenic phenotype that was found to regress with in vitro monolayer culture expansion. This had the theoretic advantage of maintaining the ability of these chondrocytes to produce a stable hyaline cartilage reparative tissue with more abundant type II collagen. Another variant of the third-generation ACI involved the use of characterized chondrocytes (characterized chondrocyte implantation), which were a subset of the chondrogenic culture-expanded population that were isolated from the monolayer culture by quantitative gene expression of certain positive and negative markers particularly developed to predict chondrocyte ability to form mature hyaline cartilage.[34] The scaffolds involved in this technique involved a 3-dimensional bovine collagen type I membrane processed in a hydrostatic bioreactor,[35,36] as well as alginate 3-dimensional beads in hydrogel-like forms.[37]

It is worth mentioning that, despite the innovation in scaffolds from the first-generation to third-generation ACI, the third-generation procedures still require a 2-stage procedure with miniarthrotomies, thus it still carries significant financial and co-morbid implications. However, all 3 generations of ACI have shown good clinical results in critical-sized OCLs of the talar dome with formation of hyaline-like cartilage at the midterm to long-term follow-up.[38,39] Due to its expense and 2-stage nature, ACIs may be best reserved as salvage procedures for large-sized OCLs (>15 mm^2) and failed MF.

AUTOLOGOUS AND ALLOGENOUS MINCED ARTICULAR CARTILAGE

In an attempt to combine the benefits of chondrocyte implantation and avoid its drawbacks, minced articular cartilage implantation was developed as a single-stage procedure that involves immediate all-arthroscopic implantation of minced autologous harvested cartilage or over-the-shelf allogenous juvenile cartilage, such as juvenile articular chondrocyte, DeNovo NT (Zimmer, Inc, Warsaw, IN, USA).

In autologous minced cartilage implantation, articular cartilage is harvested form nonweightbearing areas of the knee as with ACI and instantaneously minced in the operating theater into small fragments and loaded onto a scaffold, namely a collagen membrane or fibrin glue.

Allogenic juvenile articulated chondrocyte implants (JACIs) are done in a similar fashion after being provided commercially and stored on-shelf with a shelf life of 72 hours (**Fig. 1**). Derived from juvenile articular specimens of cadaver knees, this was based on the in vitro findings that juvenile chondrocytes exhibited a much higher anabolic activity and chondrogenic potential that superseded their counterpart adult chondrocytes, without the adverse stage of terminal chondrocyte hypertrophy.[40] The juvenile minced allogenous cartilage fragments create enough chondrocytes to treat a relatively larger OCL because finer mincing increases the total surface area and the number of exposed chondrocytes, which migrate out of the collagenous matrix and form hyaline-like cartilage.[41] The only concern for this technique is the

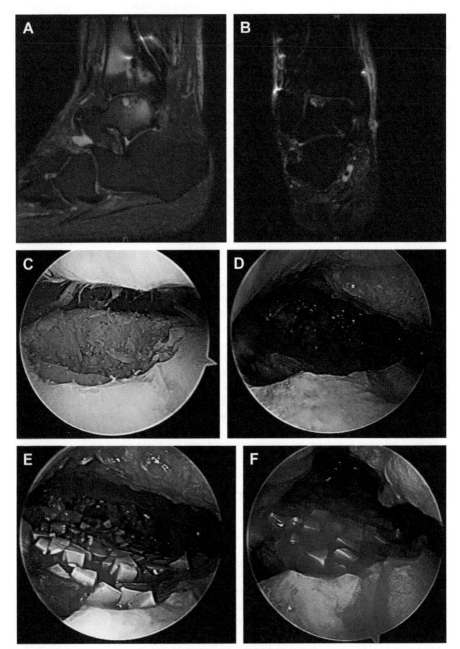

Fig. 1. Minced juvenile articulated cartilage implantation, DeNovo NT. (*A*) Short tau inversion recovery (STIR) sagittal and (*B*) coronal MRI image of an OCL of the centrolateral talar dome that was posttraumatic in origin, developing 6 months status after an ankle fracture that was managed by open reduction internal fixation. The OCL measured 15 mm × 16 mm × 10 mm deep in its widest anteroposterior, mediolateral, and craniocaudal dimensions, respectively. (*C*) Intraoperative arthroscopic image of the lesion after debridement. (*D*) Following MF, dry arthroscopy was established and the base of the OCL was filled with autologous calcaneal cancellous bone graft to the level of the chondral plate and sealed with a layer of fibrin glue. (*E*) Defect filled with juvenile articulated "minced" cartilage to the level of the surrounding cartilaginous rim. (*F*) Sealing of the surface of the DeNovo implant with fibrin glue in a "sandwich" technique.

theoretic damage induced by mincing the articular cartilage that might lead to chondrocyte death. Another concern is the amount of viable cells processed through this technique and whether these cell numbers would meet the cellular challenges of repairing the chondral lesion. However, this can be argued against by the compensatory higher metabolic activity of this cell niche. Finally, allogenic chondrocytes remain immune-privileged because they reside deep within the extra-cellular matrix, so potential immunologic reactions to the allogenic implant remain minimal.

The results of allogenous JACIs have been increasingly reported in the literature during the past few years, starting from case reports[42] to limited case series, mostly in the knee, with improved MRI signal of the repaired cartilage approximating that of normal cartilage by 2 years and hyaline-like cartilage with excellent integration on histologic examination of retrieved tissue.[43,44] In ankle OCLs, articulated juvenile chondrocyte implantation in a series of 23 subjects showed good-to-excellent results in American Orthopedic Foot and Ankle Society (AOFAS) scores postoperatively at a mean of 16-months follow-up.[45] The senior author (AH) recently reported on the largest case series of juvenile articulate chondrocyte implantation at 24-months postoperatively. This was followed up by MRI with improved magnetic resonance observation of cartilage repair tissue (MOCART) scores but persistent hypertrophy in some of the repaired OCLs, yet with significantly improved Short-Form 12 (SF-12) and Foot and Ankle Outcome Score (FAOS) compared with preoperative levels.[46] In this study, JACI was combined with bone marrow-derived aspirate concentrate (BMAC) in an attempt to obtain a more robust healing response (**Fig. 2**). This was based on in vitro evidence that coculture of BM-MSCs and chondrocytes showed an increase in chondrogenic markers.[47]

AUTOLOGOUS MATRIX-INDUCED CHONDROGENESIS

Autologous matrix-induced chondrogenesis (AMIC) is a recent modification of the MF technique. As in MF, it is a single-stage procedure in which a collagen membrane is used to collect and concentrate the mesenchymal blood clot formed after MF, instead of letting the bone marrow elements trickle from the MF holes into the joint until the mesenchymal fibrin clot forms at the base of the OCL. By collecting the MF bone marrow elements on the collagen membrane, more BM-MSCs can be captured and concentrated in the OCL to initiate a more robust healing response. AMIC has the advantage of increasing the number of recruited BM-MSCs in the chondral defect without the need for cell culture expansion, with a potential for treating larger sized defects (>10–15 mm^2) that would normally fail MF.

A second-generation AMIC procedure was also described in which the collagen membrane was saturated with BMAC obtained from the ipsilateral iliac crest intraoperatively and processed in a commercially available benchside machine. By combining AMIC and BMAC, the cellular component is significantly increased, yielding an even more robust mesenchymal cell niche that can meet the cellular challenge of repairing a critical-sized OCL.[48] Similarly, the AMIC-plus technique has also been described in which the AMIC collagen membrane is saturated with platelet-rich plasma (PRP) in an attempt to increase growth factor content of the scaffold.[49]

Due to its most recent evolution, results of AMIC in talar OCLs are limited to a handful of technical surgical notes[50,51] and small case series. The most important of which reported significant improvement in functional outcomes and MOCART scores, which demonstrated a good quality repair tissue similar to the MRI ultrastructure of the surrounding cartilage at an average of 2 year follow-up.[52] Although this seems to be promising, several studies in the knee have shown inferior reparative response on

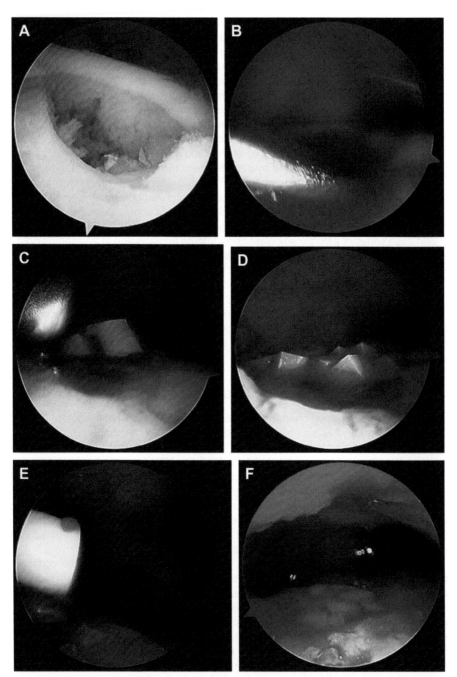

Fig. 2. JACI–BMAC. (*A*) Arthroscopic image of an OCL of the medial talar dome that measured 12 mm × 10 mm in the coronal and sagittal planes, respectively, on preoperative MRI. The lesion was half chondral and half osteochondral on intraoperative arthroscopic evaluation with only 3 mm depth at its osteochondral counterpart, which was deemed superficial enough not to warrant autologous bone grafting of the base of the defect. (*B*) After establishing dry arthroscopy, BMAC was injected into the base of the OCL via a spinal

MRI with incomplete or heterogeneous fill.[53,54] This raises the question of whether there is a sufficient concentration of the MSC niche in the AMIC membrane to support chondrogenesis and repair of critical-sized defects, with questionable long-term durability that might affect results.

BONE MARROW ASPIRATE CONCENTRATE IMPLANTATION

BM-MSCs have high chondrogenic potential and are easily accessible through aspiration of the iliac crest.[55] In Japan, initial trials using BM-MSCs were in cartilage repair of the knee through culture expansion and reimplantation in a 2-stage procedure.[56] Commercially available devices were subsequently introduced into the orthopedic field that facilitated aspiration and concentration of the bone marrow aspirate benchside in the operating room to achieve sufficient MSC numbers for a single-stage procedure without resorting to cell manipulation and culture expansion in vitro. Further testing of BMAC in treating OCLs in vivo in large animal models showed improved repair compared with MF both histologically and by MRI.[57] This set the stage for its use in the clinical setting for knee and ankle OCLs.

BMAC can be implanted on various scaffolds, including collagen membranes, hyaluronic acid–based scaffolds or as an injectable PRP-BMAC mixture[58] through an all-arthroscopic procedure. This has the potential advantages of being a simple, relatively inexpensive, and single-stage procedure that bypasses the regulatory obstacles of cell manipulation, in vitro culture expansion, and reimplantation through a second-stage procedure. The most recent injectable scaffold introduced for BMAC implantation is micronized lyophilized collagen II, tradename BioCartilage (Arthrex, Naples, FL USA), which has the merit of being easily formulated into a paste-like material after mixing with BMAC and delivered through the arthroscopic cannula into talar OCLs[59] (**Fig. 3**).

Despite being a very recent technique, results of BMAC implantation in the ankle have been promising. The Italian group which had initially reported on the procedure in 2009 for the treatment of talar OCLs[60] has recently reported their midterm outcomes of the procedure with significant improvement in postoperative AOFAS at a mean follow-up of 72 months.[61] A recent study out of the cartilage restoration group at the Hospital for Special Surgery in New York showed superior functional outcome scores and MOCART scores in talar OCLs treated by BMAC versus MF at midterm follow-up.[62]

BMAC implantation is not without its inherent limitations, one of which is an inferior MSC cellular count than those obtained by culture expansion. Once again, like other similar techniques that involve culture-free implantation of cells, these limited cellular counts might not be sufficient to meet the cellular challenges posed in healing

---

needle introduced through the arthroscopic portal in a drop-by-drop fashion to avoid overspill. This was left to clot in situ to form a bed for receiving the juvenile articulated chondrocytes. (*C*) Minced juvenile chondrocytes were delivered through the arthroscopic obturator, which was introduced via the arthroscopic portal until it perfectly overlaid the OCL. (*D*) The minced juvenile cartilage pieces were then pushed via a blunt arthroscopic trocar through the obturator into the OCL until the minced pieces were perfectly in level with the surrounding cartilaginous rim and flattened by a freer elevator to lie flush with the surface to avoid protuberance of the implant. (*E*) A dual-barrel plastic nozzle syringe was then introduced through the arthroscopic portal and fibrin glue was placed in a drop-by-drop fashion to seal the graft interface. (*F*) This was followed by further BMAC injection to the surface of the implant in a similar manner as in **Fig. 1B** and left to clot in situ for approximately 7 minutes to create the stable JACI–BMAC implant.

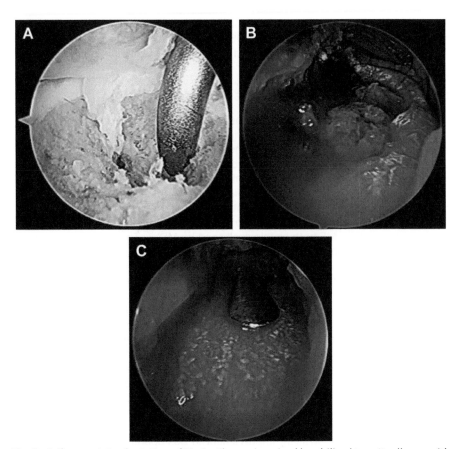

Fig. 3. Arthroscopic implantation of BioCartilage micronized lyophilized type II collagen with bone marrow aspirate concentrate (BioCartilage/BMAC). (*A*) Arthroscopic image of an OCL of the lateral talar dome measuring 12 mm × 10 mm with MF of the base of the lesion. (*B*) Filling of the base of the OCL with autologous calcaneal cancellous bone grafts to the level of the cartilaginous defect. (*C*) After establishing dry arthroscopy by draining the fluid out of the joint and thorough aspiration of any residual fluid, the micronized lyophilized type II collagen matrix mixed with autologous BMAC (Angel System; Arthrex) is introduced via an accessory arthroscopic obturator through the anteromedial arthroscopic portal to fill the chondral aspect of the OCL, then leveled flush with the surface using a freer elevator.

critical-sized OCLs. Another theoretic disadvantage of BMAC is that, despite MSC concentration, it still contains a heterogeneous cell population with other mononuclear cells, such as monocytes, that might interfere with chondrogenesis on in situ implantation by releasing cytokines and other inflammatory mediators.[63,64]

AUTOLOGOUS CULTURE-EXPANDED BONE MARROW-DERIVED MESENCHYMAL STEM CELL IMPLANTATION: THE EGYPTIAN EXPERIENCE

As previously discussed, BM-MSC was first introduced into cartilage repair as an alternative cell niche to chondrocytes, which in first-generation and second-generation ACI had exhibited low proliferative potential and dedifferentiation into fibroblast-like cells on in vitro culture expansion, and the inevitable donor site morbidity on harvest. MSCs, in contrast, had been readily available, posed no donor site morbidity, were harvested in more abundant numbers than chondrocytes, and had a more robust proliferative potential on in vitro culture expansion with excellent chondrogenic potential. The first-generation BM-MSC implant (MSCI) procedure entailed loading the culture-expanded MSCs onto a type I collagen membrane sealed by a periosteal patch and implantation via a miniarthrotomy.[56]

A second-generation MSCI was then introduced at Cairo University in Egypt in which culture-expanded stem cells were implanted on a scaffold constituting of platelet-rich fibrin glue (PR-FG) in a gel-like material that was then sealed with a periosteal patch through a miniarthrotomy. The senior author (AH) initially reported the pilot study of 5 out of 25 subjects to be treated by this second-generation MSCI in knee OCLs with improved functional knee scores and MRI findings, as well as second-look arthroscopic scores of the repair tissue.[65]

The success of the technique and encouraging results of second-generation MSCI in the knee prompted further development of this technique into an all-arthroscopic technique to treat critical-sized OCLs of the talus by injecting the BM-MSC and PR-FG mixture through the arthroscopic portal into the OCL base without the use of the periosteal patch (Video 1). This was due to the unavailability of the commercially available BMAC and PRP devices in the Middle East at that time, as well as the presence of a strong collaboration between the Orthopedic Surgery Department and the Tissue Engineering Unit of the Biochemistry Department at Cairo University, where the MSC cell cultures and PF-FG were processed. In a small case series of 16 subjects with critical-sized OCLs of the talus that averaged 3.74 cm^2 ($\pm$1.12 cm^2) and a mean short-term follow-up of 18 months, there was a slight improvement in functional outcome AOFAS postoperatively compared with preoperative scores. This improvement, however, was not statistically significant. It was attributed to several factors. First, the mean OCL size was relatively large and most OCLs were deep, with extensive edematous or cystic involvement of the underlying subchondral bone. This was managed by performing the "sandwich" technique in which autologous calcaneal bone graft was used to fill the deep OCL to the level of the subchondral bone followed by sandwiching the BM-MSC and PR-FG implants between 2 layers of fibrin glue. Despite that, the extensive and possibly persistent bony pathologic state hindered the integration of the implant. Second, the subject population was relatively older (43.1 $\pm$ 5.6 years), which might have had an effect on the chondrogenic potential of the relatively senescent MSCs. Third, the cohort size was relatively small, therefore, the study could have been underpowered to detect statistical significance in functional outcomes. Fourth, the BM-MSC and PR-FG implant was placed without a periosteal patch as was done in the knee. It is possible that the absence of the cambium layer of the periosteum, which has progenitor MSCs that can potentiate the reparative response, could have been a confounding variable in the MSCI knee study but not the talar dome OCL study.[66]

Other than this preliminary report, there are no reports in the literature on the use of BM-MSCI in talar OCLs, and most studies in the literature have reported the use of the first-generation technique in knee OCLs only.[67,68]

Disadvantages of BM-MSCI are similar to ACI in that it is a 2-stage procedure that involves ex vivo cell manipulation and culture expansion, with the potential risk of disease transmission. Moreover, the first-generation technique with the use of periosteal graft has shown potential hypertrophy of the repair tissue, with subsequent need for arthroscopic debridement and trimming of the hypertrophied reparative tissue. The most concerning element in use of culture-expanded MSCs is the potential of this cell population to go down the path of enchondral ossification with terminal hypertrophy of the MSC-derived chondrocytes, which leads to subsequent progressive ossification of the cartilaginous repair tissue. The teratogenic potential of MSCs remains merely a theoretic tentative problem and has been disputed because BM-MSCs undergo senescence, as do all other cell-lineages, and it is also negated by the safety of the BM-MSCI procedure reported at long-term follow-up.[68]

SUMMARY

Treatment of critical OCLs of the talar dome that constitute a prearthritic threat remains the holy grail of orthopedic regenerative medicine. Apart from studies showing superiority of most of the tissue engineering approaches compared with MF in critical-sized OCLs, no study has shown superiority of any modality versus another. With the orthopedic market expanding daily with new tissue engineering cartilage restoration products and ideas, it is even more difficult to compare all these different products and techniques in a solid research study that is free of commercial bias. The most recent meta-analysis examining the level of evidence in methodological studies reporting outcomes of MF, bone marrow stimulation, autologous osteochondral transplantation, osteochondral allograft transplantation, and autologous chondrocyte implantation, involved 83 studies reporting the results of 2382 subjects who underwent 2425 surgical procedures. It found no significant difference between the Coleman Methodology Score and the type of surgical technique. The meta-analysis concluded that clinical outcomes of cartilage repair of the ankle are of a low level of evidence and of poor methodologic quality.[69] This highlights the need for an international governing body to set standardized guidelines and unify all histologic, clinical, arthroscopic, and radiological outcome assessment tools for cartilage-related research. Although there have been strides on the path, steps in this field of regenerative medicine are still in their infancy.

SUPPLEMENTARY DATA

Supplementary data related to this article can be found online at http://dx.doi.org/10.1016/j.fcl.2016.01.010.

REFERENCES

1. Saxena A, Eakin C. Articular talar injuries in athletes: results of microfracture and autogenous bone graft. Am J Sports Med 2007;35(10):1680–7.
2. Berndt AL, Harty M. Transchondral fractures (osteochondritis dissecans) of the talus. J Bone Joint Surg Am 1959;41-A:988–1020.
3. Roden S, Tillegard P, Unanderscharin L. Osteochondritis dissecans and similar lesions of the talus: report of fifty-five cases with special reference to etiology and treatment. Acta Orthop Scand 1953;23(1):51–66.
4. Laffenetre O. Osteochondral lesions of the talus: current concept. Orthop Traumatol Surg Res 2010;96(5):554–66.
5. Gardiner TB. Osteochondritis dissecans in three members of one family. J Bone Joint Surg Br 1955;37-B(1):139–41.
6. Davis MW. Bilateral talar osteochondritis dissecans with lax ankle ligaments. Report of a case. J Bone Joint Surg Am 1970;52(1):168–70.
7. Stougaard J. Familial occurrence of osteochondritis dissecans. J Bone Joint Surg Br 1964;46:542–3.
8. Canale ST, Belding RH. Osteochondral lesions of the talus. J Bone Joint Surg Am 1980;62(1):97–102.

9. Bajek A, Czerwinski M, Olkowska J, et al. Does aging of mesenchymal stem cells limit their potential application in clinical practice? Aging Clin Exp Res 2012; 24(5):404–11.

10. Schimke MM, Marozin S, Lepperdinger G. Patient-specific age: the other side of the coin in advanced mesenchymal stem cell therapy. Front Physiol 2015;6:362.

11. Chuckpaiwong B, Berkson EM, Theodore GH. Microfracture for osteochondral lesions of the ankle: outcome analysis and outcome predictors of 105 cases. Arthroscopy 2008;24(1):106–12.

12. Gomoll AH, Madry H, Knutsen G, et al. The subchondral bone in articular cartilage repair: current problems in the surgical management. Knee Surg Sports Traumatol Arthrosc 2010;18(4):434–47.

13. Giannini S, Vannini F. Operative treatment of osteochondral lesions of the talar dome: current concepts review. Foot Ankle Int 2004;25(3):168–75.

14. Amendola A, Panarella L. Osteochondral lesions: medial versus lateral, persistent pain, cartilage restoration options and indications. Foot Ankle Clin 2009;14(2): 215–27.

15. van Bergen CJ, de Leeuw PA, van Dijk CN. Treatment of osteochondral defects of the talus. Rev Chir Orthop Reparatrice Appar Mot 2008;94(8 Suppl):398–408.

16. Hunt KJ, Lee AT, Lindsey DP, et al. Osteochondral lesions of the talus: effect of defect size and plantarflexion angle on ankle joint stresses. Am J Sports Med 2012;40(4):895–901.

17. Coyle CH, Izzo NJ, Chu CR. Sustained hypoxia enhances chondrocyte matrix synthesis. J Orthop Res 2009;27(6):793–9.

18. Fu WL, Zhang JY, Fu X, et al. Comparative study of the biological characteristics of mesenchymal stem cells from bone marrow and peripheral blood of rats. Tissue Eng Part A 2012;18(17–18):1793–803.

19. Knutsen G, Engebretsen L, Ludvigsen TC, et al. Autologous chondrocyte implantation compared with microfracture in the knee. A randomized trial. J Bone Joint Surg Am 2004;86-A(3):455–64.

20. Bae DK, Song SJ, Yoon KH, et al. Survival analysis of microfracture in the osteoarthritic knee-minimum 10-year follow-up. Arthroscopy 2013;29(2):244–50.

21. Kreuz PC, Erggelet C, Steinwachs MR, et al. Is microfracture of chondral defects in the knee associated with different results in patients aged 40 years or younger? Arthroscopy 2006;22(11):1180–6.

22. Mithoefer K, Williams RJ 3rd, Warren RF, et al. The microfracture technique for the treatment of articular cartilage lesions in the knee. A prospective cohort study. J Bone Joint Surg Am 2005;87(9):1911–20.

23. Anders S, Lechler P, Rackl W, et al. Fluoroscopy-guided retrograde core drilling and cancellous bone grafting in osteochondral defects of the talus. Int Orthop 2012;36(8):1635–40.

24. Zengerink M, Szerb I, Hangody L, et al. Current concepts: treatment of osteochondral ankle defects. Foot Ankle Clin 2006;11(2):331–59, vi.

25. Valderrabano V, Leumann A, Rasch H, et al. Knee-to-ankle mosaicplasty for the treatment of osteochondral lesions of the ankle joint. Am J Sports Med 2009; 37(Suppl 1):105S–11S.

26. Haleem AM, Ross KA, Smyth NA, et al. Double-plug autologous osteochondral transplantation shows equal functional outcomes compared with single-plug procedures in lesions of the talar dome: a minimum 5-year clinical follow-up. Am J Sports Med 2014;42(8):1888–95.

27. Gittens J, Haleem A, Grenier S, et al. Use of novel chitosan hydrogels for chemical tissue bonding of autologous chondral transplants. J Orthop Res 2015. [Epub ahead of print].

28. Fansa AM, Murawski CD, Imhauser CW, et al. Autologous osteochondral transplantation of the talus partially restores contact mechanics of the ankle joint. Am J Sports Med 2011;39(11):2457–65.

29. Evans PJ, Miniaci A, Hurtig MB. Manual punch versus power harvesting of osteochondral grafts. Arthroscopy 2004;20(3):306–10.

30. Redman SN, Dowthwaite GP, Thomson BM, et al. The cellular responses of articular cartilage to sharp and blunt trauma. Osteoarthritis Cartilage 2004;12(2): 106–16.

31. Wood JJ, Malek MA, Frassica FJ, et al. Autologous cultured chondrocytes: adverse events reported to the United States Food and Drug Administration. J Bone Joint Surg Am 2006;88(3):503–7.

32. Steinwachs M. New technique for cell-seeded collagen-matrix-supported autologous chondrocyte transplantation. Arthroscopy 2009;25(2):208–11.

33. Ossendorf C, Kaps C, Kreuz PC, et al. Treatment of posttraumatic and focal osteoarthritic cartilage defects of the knee with autologous polymer-based three-dimensional chondrocyte grafts: 2-year clinical results. Arthritis Res Ther 2007; 9(2):R41.

34. Saris DB, Vanlauwe J, Victor J, et al. Characterized chondrocyte implantation results in better structural repair when treating symptomatic cartilage defects of the knee in a randomized controlled trial versus microfracture. Am J Sports Med 2008;36(2):235–46.

35. Crawford DC, DeBerardino TM, Williams RJ 3rd. NeoCart, an autologous cartilage tissue implant, compared with microfracture for treatment of distal femoral cartilage lesions: an FDA phase-II prospective, randomized clinical trial after two years. J Bone Joint Surg Am 2012;94(11):979–89.

36. Crawford DC, Heveran CM, Cannon WD Jr, et al. An autologous cartilage tissue implant NeoCart for treatment of grade III chondral injury to the distal femur: prospective clinical safety trial at 2 years. Am J Sports Med 2009;37(7):1334–43.

37. Selmi TA, Verdonk P, Chambat P, et al. Autologous chondrocyte implantation in a novel alginate-agarose hydrogel: outcome at two years. J Bone Joint Surg Br 2008;90(5):597–604.

38. Kwak SK, Kern BS, Ferkel RD, et al. Autologous chondrocyte implantation of the ankle: 2- to 10-year results. Am J Sports Med 2014;42(9):2156–64.

39. Giannini S, Buda R, Ruffilli A, et al. Arthroscopic autologous chondrocyte implantation in the ankle joint. Knee Surg Sports Traumatol Arthrosc 2014;22(6):1311–9.

40. Adkisson HD, Martin JA, Amendola RL, et al. The potential of human allogeneic juvenile chondrocytes for restoration of articular cartilage. Am J Sports Med 2010; 38(7):1324–33.

41. Farr J, Yao JQ. Chondral defect repair with particulated juvenile cartilage allograft. Cartilage 2011;2(4):346–53.

42. Stevens HY, Shockley BE, Willett NJ, et al. Particulated juvenile articular cartilage implantation in the knee: a 3-year EPIC-μCT and histological examination. Cartilage 2014;5(2):74–7.

43. Farr J, Tabet SK, Margerrison E, et al. Clinical, radiographic, and histological outcomes after cartilage repair with particulated juvenile articular cartilage: a 2-year prospective study. Am J Sports Med 2014;42(6):1417–25.

44. Tompkins M, Hamann JC, Diduch DR, et al. Preliminary results of a novel single-stage cartilage restoration technique: particulated juvenile articular cartilage allograft for chondral defects of the patella. Arthroscopy 2013;29(10):1661–70.
45. Coetzee JC, Giza E, Schon LC, et al. Treatment of osteochondral lesions of the talus with particulated juvenile cartilage. Foot Ankle Int 2013;34(9):1205–11.
46. Desandis B, Haleem AM, Sofka C, et al. Juvenile allogenous articular cartilage and autologous bone marrow aspirate concentrate in the arthroscopic treatment of critical sized talar osteochondral lesions. American Orthopedic Foot and Ankle Society Annual Meeting. Long Beach (CA), July 15–18, 2015.
47. Acharya C, Adesida A, Zajac P, et al. Enhanced chondrocyte proliferation and mesenchymal stromal cells chondrogenesis in coculture pellets mediate improved cartilage formation. J Cell Physiol 2012;227(1):88–97.
48. de Girolamo L, Bertolini G, Cervellin M, et al. Treatment of chondral defects of the knee with one step matrix-assisted technique enhanced by autologous concentrated bone marrow: in vitro characterisation of mesenchymal stem cells from iliac crest and subchondral bone. Injury 2010;41(11):1172–7.
49. Dhollander AA, De Neve F, Almqvist KF, et al. Autologous matrix-induced chondrogenesis combined with platelet-rich plasma gel: technical description and a five pilot patients report. Knee Surg Sports Traumatol Arthrosc 2011;19(4): 536–42.
50. Piontek T, Bakowski P, Ciemniewska-Gorzela K, et al. Arthroscopic treatment of chondral and osteochondral defects in the ankle using the autologous matrix-induced chondrogenesis technique. Arthrosc Tech 2015;4(5):e463–9.
51. Usuelli FG, de Girolamo L, Grassi M, et al. All-arthroscopic autologous matrix-induced chondrogenesis for the treatment of osteochondral lesions of the talus. Arthrosc Tech 2015;4(3):e255–9.
52. Kubosch EJ, Erdle B, Izadpanah K, et al. Clinical outcome and T2 assessment following autologous matrix-induced chondrogenesis in osteochondral lesions of the talus. Int Orthop 2016;40(1):65–71.
53. Kusano T, Jakob RP, Gautier E, et al. Treatment of isolated chondral and osteochondral defects in the knee by autologous matrix-induced chondrogenesis (AMIC). Knee Surg Sports Traumatol Arthrosc 2012;20(10):2109–15.
54. Gille J, Schuseil E, Wimmer J, et al. Mid-term results of Autologous Matrix-Induced Chondrogenesis for treatment of focal cartilage defects in the knee. Knee Surg Sports Traumatol Arthrosc 2010;18(11):1456–64.
55. Miljkovic ND, Cooper GM, Marra KG. Chondrogenesis, bone morphogenetic protein-4 and mesenchymal stem cells. Osteoarthritis Cartilage 2008;16(10): 1121–30.
56. Wakitani S, Imoto K, Yamamoto T, et al. Human autologous culture expanded bone marrow mesenchymal cell transplantation for repair of cartilage defects in osteoarthritic knees. Osteoarthritis Cartilage 2002;10(3):199–206.
57. Fortier LA, Potter HG, Rickey EJ, et al. Concentrated bone marrow aspirate improves full-thickness cartilage repair compared with microfracture in the equine model. J Bone Joint Surg Am 2010;92(10):1927–37.
58. Steinwachs MR, Waibl B, Wopperer S, et al. Matrix-associated chondroplasty: a novel platelet-rich plasma and concentrated nucleated bone marrow cell-enhanced cartilage restoration technique. Arthrosc Tech 2014;3(2):e279–82.
59. Desai S. Surgical treatment of a tibial osteochondral defect with debridement, marrow stimulation, and micronized allograft cartilage matrix-an all-arthroscopic technique: a case report. J Foot Ankle Surg 2014;55(2):279–82.

60. Giannini S, Buda R, Vannini F, et al. One-step bone marrow-derived cell transplantation in talar osteochondral lesions. Clin Orthop Relat Res 2009;467(12): 3307–20.
61. Buda R, Vannini F, Cavallo M, et al. One-step bone marrow-derived cell transplantation in talarosteochondral lesions: mid-term results. Joints 2013;1(3):102–7.
62. Hannon CP, Ross KA, Murawski CD, et al. Arthroscopic bone marrow stimulation and concentrated bone marrow aspirate for osteochondral lesions of the talus: a case-control study of functional and magnetic resonance observation of cartilage repair tissue outcomes. Arthroscopy 2016;32(2):339–47.
63. Kubo S, Cooper GM, Matsumoto T, et al. Blocking vascular endothelial growth factor with soluble Flt-1 improves the chondrogenic potential of mouse skeletal muscle-derived stem cells. Arthritis Rheum 2009;60(1):155–65.
64. Wehling N, Palmer GD, Pilapil C, et al. Interleukin-1beta and tumor necrosis factor alpha inhibit chondrogenesis by human mesenchymal stem cells through NF-kappaB-dependent pathways. Arthritis Rheum 2009;60(3):801–12.
65. Haleem AM, Singergy AA, Sabry D, et al. The clinical use of human culture-expanded autologous bone marrow mesenchymal stem cells transplanted on platelet-rich fibrin glue in the treatment of articular cartilage defects: a pilot study and preliminary results. Cartilage 2010;1(4):253–61.
66. Gomaa MA, AbouSayed M, Haleem AM. The use of culture expanded autologous bone marrow mesenchymal stem cells in the treatment of critical-sized osteochondral lesions of the Talus Egyptian Arthroscopic Association International Congress. Cairo (Egypt), February 26–28, 2013.
67. Nejadnik H, Hui JH, Feng Choong EP, et al. Autologous bone marrow-derived mesenchymal stem cells versus autologous chondrocyte implantation: an observational cohort study. Am J Sports Med 2010;38(6):1110–6.
68. Wakitani S, Okabe T, Horibe S, et al. Safety of autologous bone marrow-derived mesenchymal stem cell transplantation for cartilage repair in 41 patients with 45 joints followed for up to 11 years and 5 months. J Tissue Eng Regen Med 2011; 5(2):146–50.
69. Pinski JM, Boakye LA, Murawski CD, et al. Low level of evidence and methodologic quality of clinical outcome studies on cartilage repair of the ankle. Arthroscopy 2016;32(1):214–22.e1.

Index

Note: Page numbers of article titles are in **boldface** type.

Foot Ankle Clin N Am 21 (2016) 421–449
http://dx.doi.org/10.1016/S1083-7515(16)30021-3
1083-7515/16/$ – see front matter

Moving?

Make sure your subscription moves with you!

To notify us of your new address, find your **Clinics Account Number** (located on your mailing label above your name), and contact customer service at:

Email: journalscustomerservice-usa@elsevier.com

800-654-2452 (subscribers in the U.S. & Canada)
314-447-8871 (subscribers outside of the U.S. & Canada)

Fax number: 314-447-8029

Elsevier Health Sciences Division
Subscription Customer Service
3251 Riverport Lane
Maryland Heights, MO 63043

*To ensure uninterrupted delivery of your subscription, please notify us at least 4 weeks in advance of move.

Printed and bound by CPI Group (UK) Ltd, Croydon, CR0 4YY

08/05/2025

01865194-0001